Simply Give Birth
A Collection of Stories

Heather Cushman-Dowdee
and Friends

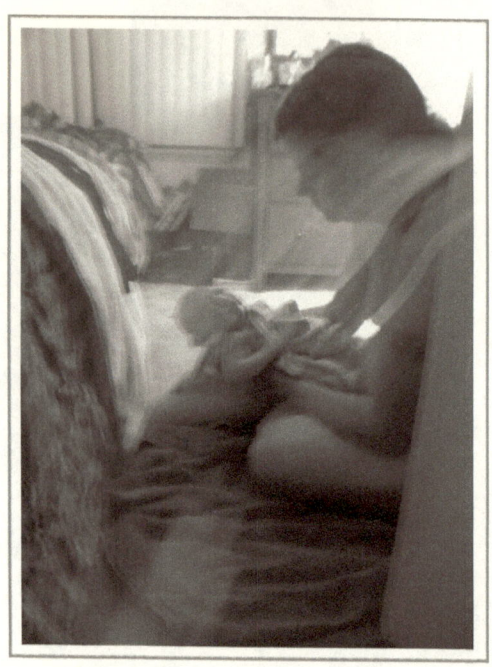

This book is dedicated to Ean, perfect in every way.

ISBN 978-0-557-13810-4
Published by Hathor! Publishing
Printed and distributed by Lulu.com or direct from the artist at
www.thecowgoddess.com or www.mama-is.com
© 2009 Heather Cushman-Dowdee all rights reserved
The artist may grant permissions but you have to ask first
hathor@thecowgoddess,com

...And Friends

T he idea for the book *Simply Give Birth* came to me a couple of years ago, as most of my ideas come to me, while breastfeeding. This particular day was unexceptional, except that I happened to sit down to nurse a sleepy baby and forgot to grab my book first. So I fished around in a drawer beside the chair and unearthed a stack of *The New Nativity* — a quarterly collection of unassisted birth stories. Lo and behold, that's when and where I read *Fiery's Birth Story* by Poppy Street-Heywood. Poppy begins her birth story with, "45 weeks and 4 days. That's how long Fiery took to enter the crazy world outside my body." Then casually, almost as if it were not the most important thing in the world, describes her birth that was long overdue and yet, somehow didn't seem to cause her any fear or complaint. She just simply gives birth. Right there in the bathroom, just like it was any other day. And then, that's when she got me with this line: "My other two births were not medically necessary c-sections before labor..." and I was hooked. I wanted to know more! How had she the composure? How had she the faith? The spirit? Then like a fisher pulling in the big marlin she passes the pen to her husband and lets him tell his side of the story too. Humorous, witty, matter-of-fact, he claims that he "wasn't worried at all." I believed him. And my first thought was that this story needed to get out there into the world.

I contacted the editor of *The New Nativity*, and she helped me get in touch with Poppy. I asked her for permission to use her story. For what, I had no idea, but something, something…fast forward a few months later and I'm asked to speak at The Trust Birth Conference and an idea came to me, that for too long the other story, the drama, and pain and horrifyingly out-of-control helplessness, has been the predominant tale. It's time for that story to go the way of dinosaurs. There's a new way to tell our birth stories, a simple way, with humor and spirit and matter-of-fact exuberance, and that if we collect these types of stories and spread them out into the world, we'll be spreading the idea that birth is a funny, crazy, everyday, yet still life-changing to our very core, experience. Because it is all that. And more.

Choosing the Stories

I put out a call on my website for birth stories in the beginning of 2007, that read like this:

Calling for Birth Stories!

If you have a birth story (preferably unassisted, but if it's assisted it shouldn't focus too much on the midwife—not that she's not totally *awesome*, please don't misunderstand, I *love* midwives! I'm looking for birth stories that focus on the mother, the baby and the birth process.) Please send it in to be included in the next Hathor book (I'm too poor to pay you, but will happily give you a couple of the books and my undying gratitude!) Plus, you'll be in print! My friend, Gurumama (Mara Donahoe), is going to be editing the book so I'll be passing the stories along to her and she'll be in touch about whether they'll be included or not...Please forward this widely!

Here's what you can do to make the birth story exactly what I'm looking for:

1. Remove the paragraphs where you're making your decision to birth at home or birth unassisted. For instance, in my birth story of Gwyneth Kai, I'm going to remove the first paragraph where I blather on about wanting a birth that was free of interventions. For the sake of argument, let's agree that the audience for this book already *wants* a birth that's free of interventions. Let's *assume* we live in a world where *all* women want no interventions. It's a given. How would you start your birth story then...probably at the first contraction, huh? Okay, start there.

2. If you're telling an unassisted birth story or an assisted birth story, let's just call it a birth. Take out all the qualifiers and just birth that baby!

3. Fear is fine, but how 'bout a little bit about how you *rise above* the fear? And don't forget to include those moments when you weren't afraid. I like to read birth stories where the laboring mother "just knew" what to do. It comforts me, and when I gave birth the third time I was able to tune into my instincts because I had read so many birth stories by women who *just knew.*
    And...

4. If you think your birth story can do all of this, but it includes an intervention anyway heck, send it in. Interventions happen, as do transfers. It's how we *feel* (and write) about them that matters. Can your birth story tell how you transferred to the hospital and delivered your breech baby into the hands of some strange doctor, but still, wow! Isn't birth great and wouldn't you do it again?

So, that's what I'm looking for…please send them in!

This request was answered by about a hundred mothers with wondrous stories, courageous stories, fantastical stories and then *oh*, how to pick? First, in the spirit of true delegation I forwarded all the birth stories to Mara to read because that seemed the best way. But then as I was opening the emails I started to sort of skim them and then to read them. Then, succumbing to some kind of birth-story fever, you could find me carrying around a big pink folder full of printed birth stories and plopping myself down on a picnic blanket in my local playground and just reading. I read birth stories on the beach, in the car, everywhere I could. They were, every one of them so good that I had trouble getting them out of my mind. In the end I picked about 30 stories. They are, for the most part, unassisted, though it was really their tone that made me choose them. They seem to focus on the birth most of all and leave the cast of other characters in the wings, as they should be. The problem was that in picking 30, it meant that I wasn't choosing 70+ birth stories and these were all really good too! So I thought I'd include a few highlights so that you can see what I mean.

For instance, in Thalea's Birth Story by Jessica, I was on the edge of my seat with

> "I did what I could to not push too hard. Finally, her head appeared, for the first time in four births I was able to reach down and feel my baby as she was coming out."

Sing it sister, my soul cried! Then Leigh Steele writing in *Birth Story: Indigo Sol* had me in full anticipation with

> "The overwhelming feeling of spontaneous pushing coupled with active pushing was new to me, something I was unable to experience with Kaia's birth. I had been anxiously looking forward to this part and now I seemed to be drowning in the sounds and intense feelings associated with it. I couldn't get over how forceful it was, how the bearing down feeling overtook my body and I had no control. And while I added extra pushing efforts, my body instinctively did most of the

work. No "breathing this baby out" like I'd hoped to do! Nope, this was raw and primal, rough and tumble, a feeling so huge and powerful for my small body. My body has been overcome."

And then laughing along with

"I begin to get my wish and can see a bit of 'baby' in the mirror and the video camera screen. The yellowish-whitish color is shocking to me for some reason and I ask 'what is it?' I hear laughs and something like "Your baby. It's a butt crack, a tiny little butt crack!" My silly breech babies, I think, and this thought lightens the mood momentarily. At this point, the feeling of stretching is unlike anything I could have imagined. It doesn't burn, it doesn't really 'hurt' it's just so damn *intense* (the only word I can come up with to describe the entire labor). With prompting, I reach down and touch my baby with one of my fingers and gently rub her bum, glorious, glorious emotion! Smooth and soft, wet and perfect. I cannot believe the time is almost here to greet her."

In many of the stories there was a sense of humor, an acknowledgement that birth is weird, wacky and uncertain. Keri West says in *Birth Story: Maya*

"My husband massaged my back, while I ate candy and we whiled away the afternoon.

Around 5 p.m. things started to get pretty intense. I was hot and my feelings of introspective busy-ness had upgraded to a *need something to do* something. I was wandering around the room trying the birth ball, the shower, and the bed; and alternately chanting "ba-by, ba-by" and whining "I don't want to dooOOoooo this anymore" My mom and husband walked on either side of me and held me up when contractions melted my knees. Maya was crowning but she was coming no further. Each push she seemed to retreat a little more. I was starting to get tired but Maya's heartbeat was strong and steady throughout. Finally we found the right position on the bed, my mom holding my left knee and my husband holding the right knee. The midwives knotted a bed sheet and I pulled against them like it was tug-of-war while my family pushed against me. Their energy was my energy. We all moved in this amazing muscular wave and POW! Maya shot out so fast the midwife had to dive to catch her at the end of the bed!"

There is a consensus that birthing pools, while giving your dearest husband something to do, and allowing you the opportunity to take the giant extra load of weight you're carrying off your legs/feet/ass, really only add to the hilarity. Talitha Sherman tells in *Good Birth Story*

"Our pool story, or, a comedy of errors: I hadn't wanted the pool to begin with. I didn't (and still don't) like the idea of soaking in my own filth or birth fluids. But my midwife insisted that there was nothing more soothing than water in labor, so we set it up on faith. What a disaster! First of all, we had no pump. Dan and the midwife took turns blowing up the pool. They both got lightheaded and it took forever. Then they set up the hose from outside to fill the pool with cool water. My brilliant cat decided to jump over the hose, but she didn't quite make it. She ended up knocking it out of the pool and setting it whipping around the living room soaking everything including me, my lunch, and the cat. I was so upset! I started to cry and went upstairs to change and dry off. Downstairs, all my old towels that I had set aside for the birth were being used to clean up the water. My mother-in-law arrived at some point in all this water fun and started helping out with cleanup. Next, my midwife went into our closet to hook the hose up to the water heater and gashed her forehead open on the sloping ceiling in the closet. So Dan was drying the furniture, my MIL was giving first aid to the midwife, I was alone upstairs having contractions, and the cat was in the backyard feeling insulted. When the water heater hookup finally happened, out gushed years of silt and debris from the bottom of the water heater. So, after all that, my three assistants ended up bailing filthy water into our small patio yard, flooding it, and I had no birth pool, which I didn't want to begin with. We affectionately refer to this water misadventure as Hurricane Fran. (It was the year Hurricane Fran struck and our midwife is named Fran.)

Anyway, after that, all I had to do was give birth."

All she had to do, indeed! Heather Sutton makes it seem as easy as all that in *My Last Two Births Were Incredible*

"I never even knew I was in transition with him. When the midwife showed up, I was lying on the floor curled in a fetal position, gripping the edge of the coffee table for all I was worth. She decided to check me and told me I was at ten centimeters. I was shocked. I slid into my pool and...waited for an hour to have an urge to push. Then, once I plopped onto my bottom, he was ready to go! The most incredible feeling in the world was to hold this tiny little person and realize I'd birthed him, in the presence of his Daddy and big sister, with no drugs, no tears, no screams for me to "Push!" It was quiet, gentle, loving, dark, and soothing. We sat in the cooling water for an hour and just gazed at each other. I was hooked on birth for the first time in five births."

And then with her next birth she says

"I was on my hands and knees staring into two inches of water in my birth pool (blown up this time by a plug-in air compressor) when I realized the little man was on his way. I called out to my husband that the baby was coming. He called back "Yes, Honey, I know." I very calmly told him, "No, Honey, the baby is coming *now*." By the time he made it from our kitchen sink to the birthing pool (maybe ten feet) our son was crowning. He came into the world as peacefully and calmly as I can imagine, with his Daddy catching him, his big sister bringing blankets and scissors and the midwife still a quarter mile away."

12

See how hard it was to pick from these awesome stories? Every one of them is a life-changing, life-affirming event, and I feel ever more goddess-like that I was given the opportunity to bask in them.

In the end most of the stories I chose were unassisted. I wanted stories that were without the intrusion of an outer voice, and followed the internal guidance of the mother alone. I found them, a *lot* of them, and then I found this one too, *Birth Story* by Teresa Stire, about a mother who followed her internal guidance while ignoring and all but barricading herself off from the outer voices. I'm not going to reprint the whole story, but here are some highlights:

> "Having already had three Cesareans, the last one being a homebirth transport, I was at a loss for what to do in the way of birth plans with this pregnancy. What I really was hoping for was to find someone who could take a look at my medical records with me (including mention of my 'markedly thin lower uterine segment', my 'narrow pubic arch', my 'single-sutured uterine closure', my 'incisional hernia' and whatever else labels I had worried myself about) and talk with me about the risks and the benefits of having another Cesarean vs. having a homebirth. I spent a lot of hours praying and asking God to please instill in me the wisdom to know what His will was for this birth and this baby. I quickly ruled out a hospital VBAC, knowing that it wasn't an environment where I could labor effectively or feel comfortable in; therefore, I really wasn't interested in pursuing it as an option. This left me with the options of having another Cesarean or birthing my baby at home. I called around, talked to various midwives, and got a referral to a direct-entry midwife who had gone back to osteopathic school to become a doctor, opened her own birth center, and still did home births as well (along with having a family practice). She was in a very rural community three hours away and I decided to make the trek down to see her. The minute I met her, it was an instant "click," and I knew that I wanted her involved in my birth in some capacity. As she listened to the stories of my previous Cesareans, she said to me

with tears in her eyes, 'There is nothing wrong with your pelvis, your uterus, or any other part of your body. What you need is to be left alone while you labor. You need to feel free to do whatever you need to do without anyone watching you. Your assignment is to figure out what you need in order to feel uninhibited and to birth this baby.'"

Okay, remember that quote later!

> "I thought a lot about that in the subsequent months, and I came to realize that she had hit the nail on the head, and what I needed in order to feel safe was to be left alone to do the work of labor, to not feel watched, or timed, or scrutinized in any way…"

Unfortunately (as if to test her mettle) Teresa's water broke and then not much of anything happened for about eleven days, but she hung in there and continued to wait patiently until

> "Saturday, April 14 rolled around, and while it seemed to be much like the previous eleven days, there was also something distinctly different about it, about me, that day. The peace I'd been feeling for the previous weeks seemed to have dissipated; I was *cranky*! I was irrational, unreasonable, and just beside myself. I was thoroughly finished with being pregnant, was certain that this baby was just not going to come out without being cut out, and that I was surely broken. As Clare tried to convince me otherwise, and coax me onto the treadmill, or into some other sort of movement or motion to elevate my mood, I lost it. I told her how 'I have done everything within my power to get this baby into a good position and try to get it to want to be born. I have done chiropractic and acupuncture every week for the past nine months. I have meditated, I have visualized, I've talked to the baby, I've exercised faithfully, I've done Optimum Fetal Positioning so much my knees are bruised, I just can't do anymore. I can't listen to you blaming me for not doing enough! I have had it. I am *done*! I am just *done*! Why

14

can't you just admit that I am *broken*? It is time for me to just throw in the towel and admit that my body is broken! My pelvis is messed up and I can't birth this baby.' And with that I stomped off in a rage."

Luckily this mood passes and she finds the peace she needed again

"It was a beautiful spring night, so I decided to go out on the front porch. I wrapped up in a blanket on the wicker furniture. I would stand up during a contraction and move my hips around in large circles or figure eight's, and turn up the 'labor music' and breathe and moan as I felt the surge overtake me. Then between the contractions, I would turn the music off and sit quietly, enjoying the sound of the crickets and the brightness of the moon. I think it was at some point during my time outside that I realized 'I think I might actually be in labor this time. It's been over four hours now, and things do not seem to be going away, but getting more intense.' As soon as that thought entered my mind, an instant excitement filled the air, and I was almost giddy with anticipation. Here I was in the stillness of the night, laboring alone in peace and working beautifully through each of these contractions! It was as if I was dreaming and I started to cry and think to myself, 'I have waited for so many years for this moment and it's finally here!'

As I stepped up the step to go back inside, I could literally feel the baby's head moving down lower into my pelvis and feel my pelvic bones slowly stretching apart. The contractions became even more intense and immediately went to about three minutes apart."

So she did what any laboring woman would do, especially one who knew she needed to be left alone, she fit her body into a small space in between the bed and the wall:

"Over in the corner by my side of the bed, in a space so small that Steve could barely fit in there with me. But that is where I

15

felt comfortable and secure."

And when the midwife showed up?

> "It was strange really, looking back. Before the midwife
> arrived, I had no conscious awareness of anyone else in the
> room, or even the world. I had this concentrated belief that this
> was all within me, I was the *only* one who could do this job.
> But then when she arrived, I began to get sidetracked and a bit
> panicky. I started looking to her to save me or something,
> asking her 'Am I okay? Is everything all right?' to which she
> would reply, 'Do you think you're okay? Do you feel like
> every thing's all right?' and when I would ask, "What if I need
> to go to the hospital?" she would reply "Do you feel like you
> need to go to the hospital?" and unfailingly turn all of my
> doubts and fears back onto me, and force me to go even deeper
> within myself and trust my instincts, to which I would
> immediately get an answer, 'Of course I'm okay. I am birthing
> my baby' or 'No, I don't need to go to the hospital. Drugs
> sound mighty nice right now, but I am doing just fine without
> them.'"

Then the birth:

> "After that contraction, the midwife asked if I would be willing
> to move out to the middle of the room, or into the birthing tub,
> or somewhere else (she is seeing that birth is imminent; I am
> not seeing it). 'No, I like it here. I want to stay here.' Steve
> then picked up the stool I'd been leaning on and said, 'Come
> on, T. We'll go to my side of the bed. There's more room over
> there.' And so up I go. As I got halfway around the bed, I have
> a contraction in the middle of the room. It's terrible, painful,
> scary! I feel so exposed and vulnerable! As soon as it ends, I
> rushed back into a corner on his side of the bed (which does
> have more space, but not much), I 'assume the position' that I
> have become so fond of, and turned my back to everyone else
> in the room. About that time, this unbelievable, out-of-

nowhere, extraterrestrial-feeling compulsion invades every cell of my body and I feel every single inch of myself start to push and heave and thrust and work and groan. What on earth? And then a small voice inside my head says, 'Hey, I wonder if I'm pushing?' (Okay…so I'm a bit slow to figure things out.)

I put my hand down and reach inside and I feel the most indescribable, inexpressible, utterly beyond words sensation that my fingertips have ever felt. There it was, no more than an inch or two inside my body, my baby's head. My. Baby's. Head. It was at that moment that I believed, wholly believed, for the first time since the scalpel made its first cut eleven years earlier, that I was going to give birth to my baby. I was capable, my body was perfectly made, my pelvis was adequate, my uterus was strong, and my baby was about to be born. I was suspended in this hazy, quasi-reality…the moment froze and a flood of emotions just rolled over me. I was caught between wanting to just stop everything right there and savor this most miraculous experience and wanting to push with everything I had in me to get this baby out here and kiss his or her beautiful face and touch that squishy head with my chin and my lips and hold him or her close to me.

Eventually the latter won out and I started pushing with another contraction, all the while thinking, 'Well, I am almost 100% sure this baby is going to come out my butt. But there is not a thing I can do about it, but get it out.' I was remembering other women's similar experiences on the ICAN (International Cesarean Awareness Network) list about pushing being 'shockingly rectal' or something like that, and that gave me some comfort, but mostly I just felt like I didn't really care if it did decide to come out my butt. Again, I put my hand down there and felt that amazing baby head, and someone asks, 'What are you doing? Why are you putting your hand down there?' 'Because, there is a baby right there. It's about to be born.' At this proclamation, the scurrying began, grabbing cameras and blankets and getting in position to hopefully get a hand on this baby, although as the midwife said, this had to have been the most difficult position for her to get in there and catch the baby, and to which I replied, 'I really was unconcerned with your comfort or ease at that point.'

I laid my head down and rested and maybe even dozed for a few minutes while waiting for the next contraction. It was so quiet and so surreal to me right then. There was nowhere else in the world I would want to be, nowhere in the world was anything as important going on as this undertaking right here. As the contraction began to build, I raised my head, gathered up every ounce of anything I had and gave a huge push and felt this incredible sensation of the slippery, squishy head sliding through and out of my body, followed by the body. I looked up in my foggy haze and asked, 'What do I do now?' to which my darling husband quickly replies, '*Don't sit down!*'…The baby was right under me. The midwife calmly unwrapped the cord from his neck and handed him to me. '6:56 a.m.' Clare announced. So he was born after about eight and a half hours of active labor, twenty or so total hours of some intense prodromal labor, and nearly two weeks of ruptured membranes. I am *so* thankful that it happened the way that it did and I got a lot of the 'work' out of the way as I went along. And also so thankful that I never had a vaginal exam so I never knew whether to be excited, frustrated, discouraged, etc., other than what my body told me to be.

I took him in my arms and the first thing I did was to thank him, 'Thank you, thank you so much for doing this with me baby.' Then I turned to my husband and I have never seen such a look of awe and admiration and love in anyone's eyes as I did in his at that moment, which probably mirrored what he saw in mine. We just sat there for a moment and looked into each other's eyes as I proclaimed, 'We *did it!* I did it! I just pushed a baby out of my vagina. I really did it! I just can't believe I did it!' "

See? I wasn't even going to print this story in its entirety, but here it is in its entirety. Because this story is so wonderful, so marvelous, and so perfect. Just like all the birth stories, chosen or not, it proves what can be done. We can birth our babies *and* relish it too. We're not stoic, or fanatical, we're mothers doing what mothers have always done, giving birth; with grace and spirit, and chutzpah, and moxie. These are the kinds of stories that helped me when I was in labor with my last child and I hope these stories, the ones that I chose to fill the book and the ones that I excerpted here, help you when you're on your way to that wondrous rite of passage, birth. There are many, many, many, inspiring stories about birth out there in the world; and it's the inspiring ones that we should share.

The mothers who submitted their stories to my safekeeping did share; they shared their grief, their passions, their exaltation, and their fears. It takes massive courage to write about this most personal of moments with such candor and intensity and then be willing to share it with the likes of me. Now we're sharing them with you, dear reader. I am so grateful that I got to read them, every single one.

Love,
Heather Cushman-Dowdee

45 Weeks and 4 days: Unassisted Birth after Two C-sections
Poppy Street-Hayward

I started having contractions at about 7 a.m. My mom picked me up around 9 a.m. for a big day of shopping that I had been promising myself for months. I was having contractions every few minutes the whole day. My mom said (around 2 p.m.) that they seemed about five minutes apart. I was unimpressed, as they had been the same way, all day, the day before — only to go away at night. And two days before that, same thing. And even a few weeks before *that*. So I was fully prepared for them to go away again any time.

When I got home at about 6 p.m., I was still having them, and decided to time a few. They were like three minutes or so apart. I never timed again after that. Around 10 p.m., I was puking and having lots of bloody show, so I figured this was probably the real thing at last. I called my friend Molly and told her it was probably going to be tonight and asked her to inform the Internet for me. Then I went back in the bathroom to labor.

I labored alone in the bathroom because it was nice and dark and private. My contractions were heavy and strong. My uterus is made of steel, piss, and vinegar. I didn't really try to do anything to make them more bearable, I just went with them. Around midnight my uterus started pushing.

I was making loud low noises the whole time, though my husband says it wasn't really that loud. At 12:30 I poked my head out and asked my husband what time it was. He told me and I said, "Okay, I can do this until 6 a.m." Not that I had a plan for what would happen at 6 a.m.!

My uterus continued its pushing for a long time. With each contraction I would have three long hard pushes with nary a pause between them. At one point I felt inside my vagina (up until this point I didn't go inside myself at all) and I could feel her head way up there. I opened the door and told Steve (my husband) that the baby was coming and to come in the bathroom with me. For most of my pushing I was either squatting, kneeling, or on my hands and knees up to this point. I decided to go with hands and knees for delivery just to avoid any chance of stuck shoulders. This meant my husband would do the baby catching, and I wouldn't be having the solo birth I had planned. I really didn't care at the time, and, in retrospect, I'm glad he was able to participate in such a cool event. Anyway...

So he came in and sat behind me. I felt inside myself a few more times to feel the baby descending and made him feel too. He said he was scared to put his fingers in me, and I told him, "Do it!" I felt that it would prepare him for her birth, to feel her coming. About fifteen minutes after I called him in the bathroom, she began to crown. I could hear her sputter as she opened her mouth a bit and wiggled around. I asked Steve if she had any hair, he said yes, lots of it. I didn't like not being able to see, but I trusted him. I asked if there was cord around her neck, and reminded him that if he couldn't see it not to feel for it. He couldn't see cord until her shoulders were coming out, and he said it was loose and he unwound it. Then he caught her!

I sat back and picked her up. She started crying pretty quickly, and continued crying for an hour. She came out in a flood of muddy meconium. I made my husband get the towel full of meconium out of the garbage the next day so I could see it, since it was dark in the bathroom and I missed it at the time. She had poop in her hair, ears, and all in her toes, and she was beautiful, looking just as I had pictured her.

Probably about ten minutes after she was born, her placenta came out whole and with no significant signs of aging. It seemed a little small, compared to other placentas I've seen. Steve picked it up and put it in the big bowl I had handy, and it waited in the freezer for a spring burial.

She didn't nurse for over an hour, she was screaming so much, poor baby. I think she was half asleep when she was born, and I woke her up rubbing her and moving her around to make sure she was okay. That part was unexpected, but it's all good. She hasn't cried at all since she was 3 days old, so I'm not complaining! I'm in love with this baby I waited so long for. I have no regrets about doing my own prenatal care, not inducing myself in any way, or about my labor and unassisted birth. Everything was perfect, and I'd never do it any other way!

My other two births were c-sections, which were not medically necessary. The c-sections occurred before labor, and my babies were five pounds and a six pounds. I have no doubt that those pregnancies would have been longer, resulting in bigger, healthier babies, had they been left to complete. Fiery weighed in at 10 pounds 7 ounces.

My husband, the comedian, has this to add to my story:

Everything I knew about having a baby had to do with a hospital. When our last daughter, Echo, was born in the hospital, I didn't think anything of it, but Poppy was voicing many of the problems she had with the way things were handled. When Poppy first told me she wanted to have a home birth with the next child I paid little attention to her mad ramblings. Then I got her pregnant and I realized she was only going to get crazier over the next couple months so I didn't have much time to figure out what was going on and talk some sense into her. Poppy has always been very good at persuading me to do things I don't want to do (insert joke here) but I didn't want to follow along blindly when it came to something as important as our baby. I wanted to know about all the things that could go wrong. I, of course, had the most questions right at the beginning. Some are very predictable: what to do if the cord is around the neck or if the baby doesn't start to breathe on it's own—or how to handle unexpected mutant powers (hope hope). I had more and more questions over the next couple of months, many of which came from other people whom I had spoken to about having a homebirth. Poppy answered all of my questions, and we looked up many different topics and sources on the Internet until I was satisfied with the answers and felt okay.

Fast forward a couple months. I am feeling much better about this whole thing. I really see how a simple thing like having a baby in our society has gotten out of hand. The questions people were asking me and the worst-case scenarios they were presenting seemed ridiculous. Yet some of these questions were the same ones I had asked months earlier. Now, at this point, if I were reading this, I would think, "This guy is brainwashed." All I can say about that is now that I've watched the whole process, it all makes sense. My wife was very conscious about what was going on with the baby and all of her prenatal care, so it's not like you just go from pregnant to baby without knowing how things are developing.

Fast forward another couple of months. Poppy is more than one month overdue and retaining water like a sponge. Even though this was getting pretty rough for Poppy, the concern was only for her comfort not her safety. Everything was fine, everything was checking out. As I stated earlier, Poppy has talked me into a lot of things that I have been uneasy about the whole time. Like that hitchhiker we killed. But this was different. I wasn't worried at all. I was eager to see the baby and wondering what it would be like to see all of it happen for the first time, but that was it. The previous c-sections didn't matter to me either. At this point I was confident that everything was going to turn out fine. Then the payoff. Poppy calls me in the bathroom where she been pushing for, I think about an hour and a half. I'm only in there 20 minutes when I can already see the baby's head coming out. Little closed eyes then nose and mouth. Poppy asked me to check for the cord being too tight around the neck. I looked at it, no problems. Then, *pop*, here comes the baby all splishy and splashy and I caught her. That's right, first try. Now my wife can never call me useless again. There is nothing like this experience. It made me feel proud of my wife, proud of myself, proud of the baby and proud of my other two kids who were asleep during the whole thing. I didn't really feel proud of the dog, though. (She didn't do anything.) I feel very grateful to my wife, Poppy, for making this whole thing possible.

The Birth Story of Isobel Josephine
Andi Starr

Forty weeks, two days, according to my "dates". It had been a long day. Sinjin (my two-year-old boy) and I decided to head to bed around 11 p.m. We read a story, I turned off the light, said goodnight and rolled over........*pop!* It felt like the baby had landed a hell of a punch, but I didn't think anything more of it. I'd had the same sensation the night before, and nothing had come of it. I rolled over again, trying to get comfortable, and fluid gushed out. My waters had broken.

Now, if you can, imagine a woman roughly the size of a beached whale, squeezing her legs together as tightly as she can and tip-toeing to the bathroom, so as not to sploosh all over the carpet of the apartment.

I climbed into the tub and let go. Fluid went everywhere. It was clear, flecked with vernix, so all looked well. However, I kept leaking. The baby's head wasn't acting like a cork for some reason, so I quick checked to make sure there was no cord prolapse. I didn't feel anything, but suddenly got the urge to go to the bathroom. No contractions yet, though.

I made my way out to the living room and found the phone. My husband, Corey, worked nights at the time and had just gotten to work when I called. I then called my mom and my friend, Shell. Mom arrived first, then Shell, then Corey. About fifteen minutes had passed and contractions had started, so I knew we would have a baby by morning.

Sinjin was running around, tired and cranky, but excited. He knew something was happening, but he was just so exhausted he couldn't see straight, so Corey took him to bed. They both fell asleep, which was fine with me. I knew I didn't really want him around while I was laboring. Shell, Mom and I stayed out in the living room. Coffee was brewed. Some food was made. They chatted. I walked up and down the hall, stopping every few minutes to sit on the toilet. The whole time I kept leaking fluid. I had the feeling something was up, but didn't feel that it was any sort of complication, so I just pushed it to the back of my mind.

Labor progressed easily and fairly quickly. We never watched the clock or timed contractions, and I never checked my cervix. I showered, walked around, sat on the birth ball, had a bath, walked some more. Before labor, I had been looking forward to being able to eat and drink as I pleased, but when the time came, I had no appetite. So I tried my best to keep drinking water and went about my business.

I don't know what time I entered transition, but I do remember the contractions getting stronger. I laid down on the couch, wanting nothing more than to doze off for a while. I started feeling spacey and restless. I wasn't comfortable, no matter what position I tried. I ended up on my knees, leaning over the birth ball, rocking back and forth. I heard myself start moaning and growling and for a split-second thought, "Here it comes"…

The urge to push hit like a freight train, and I leaned back onto my legs, unable to control it. I had to push. I wasn't even able to form a coherent thought at this time. My mind had been taken over by instinct. All I knew was "push" and "rest."

My mother, who had had a c-section with me, her only child, had up to this point been fairly calm. For whatever reason, though, when I started growling and pushing, she decided she must hug me during every contraction. I somehow managed not to throw her across the room and ignored the fact that I was being smothered. While I had managed to lay out some sheets and towels during labor, I'd forgotten to put out anything more absorbent. So Shell managed to put chux pads and a couple more sheets under me using some sleight of hand.

I could feel the baby moving down, then being sucked back up. Turtling, I thought. No big deal, just keep going. Again, the feeling hit me that something was a little off, and that this was going to hurt and I was just going to have to summon up everything I had to get the baby down and out…

So I growled, and I pushed. By this time, Corey had woken up and was sitting in the corner. Sinjin stayed asleep. Everyone sat back, watching, as I felt the baby come down and start crowning. Shell was behind me, waiting. I had asked her to catch the baby. She was telling me "almost here"….and then I felt it. I hadn't felt it with Sinjin, so I wasn't prepared for the ring of fire. Behind the burning white hot pain, the thought ran through my mind, just once, that maybe this unassisted birth thing had been a bad idea….and then I had to push again. My hand flew down to slow the crowning and let the tissue stretch. But it felt like I was going to split up the front, and rational thought flew out the window. After that contraction and before the next, I went into panic mode. My mind was racing and my breathing became rapid. I knew I needed to do something…

It took a moment before my head cleared long enough to communicate to the rest of me "change position." At the exact same moment, I heard Shell behind me "Do you need to move? What do you want us to do?" I told her to grab the couch cushions and pile them up off to the side. I told Mom to get behind the cushions. In one movement, I flipped over into a semi-sitting/squatting position, leaned back, and with the next contraction, pushed with everything I had. The baby's head popped through, and the poor thing started crying right then! I felt the baby corkscrew, and the shoulders and legs came tumbling out, into Shell's hands. The baby was crying loudly and pinked up to a healthy all-over rosy red in seconds. Shell passed this slippery, crying creature to me. The cord was extremely short and I couldn't even get the baby to the breast without it being pulled. So I sat holding this new little person on my stomach, and I hushed and cooed, put a towel around us and spoke softly. The baby started to settle down a bit, and Shell asked "So, what do we have, Mama?" I realized I hadn't looked to see yet…

One quick glance and I announced "It's a girl! Isobel!" and the room cheered. We cut the cord soon after it stopped pulsating. It was too short for either one of us to get comfortable, and the placenta hadn't made an appearance yet. Once that was done, Izzy settled down and took in her surroundings. We checked the clock…4:40 a.m.

Izzy didn't want to nurse right away, so Mom and Corey made their introductions while my body birthed the placenta. We placed it in a plastic container, and I went and took a quick bath to clean up since I was covered in blood, while mom and Shell weighed and measured Izzy. She was so calm during that time, perfectly content to look around at her new world.

Afterwards, we settled in on the couch for our first nursing, while everyone else cleaned up. I was bruised, but no tears. That's when Shell told me…that nagging feeling I'd had that something was off….Izzy had presented with a nuchal hand. Her little fist had been balled up on the side of her face, next to her temple.

Izzy was born at home, unassisted, on May 17, 2006, at roughly 4:40 a.m., weighing in at 9 pounds 11 ounces, 22 inches long, with a 14-inch head and a nuchal hand. And I can't wait to have another!

The Birth of Solomon
Erika Devine

The pains started.

I smiled. I was going to meet you, my son, at last after nine months of sickness and waiting, waiting, waiting.

I paced my home. The pains got stronger and more demanding. I walked.

Day turned to night and I was burying my face in cushions and moaning muffled sounds.

Your father went to bed. He knew it was going to be a long time yet.

The pain subsided, came less often, less urgently.

Day came. I lay in the bath, too tired to do anything but feel my body's shivers. I slept a little in the water, waking with each contraction. I was entering a dream like state, almost ecstatic; the pain was a long way away from me, down a long tunnel.

Somehow night came again.

I started to worry. This was going to be a long labor but I was not going to lie down and give up, I was going to walk every step.

I decided to take control.

Midnight. The house was quiet, the lights down low. I took out my drum. I lay some artifacts before me: Painted stones, a necklace of beads, a vial of arnica, an image of the Goddess, a band of green ribbon. These things were given to me by my powerful sisters, my friends, at my Mother Blessing.

I tapped out a rhythm. I knew you could hear it inside of me. I drummed a beat that came from beyond this age of needles, white rooms and separation. It came from my heart, my ancient heart. It came from my mother and her mother before her.

The pains grew stronger and more urgent.

I needed others to drum the beat for me now but I was alone so I put music on so that I could dance. In another time, another life, my sisters would have made the music on their drums and with their song but this was now and so the music came through a machine.

I danced.

You danced inside me and slipped further into place.

The pain was swift and strong but I owned it now.

When the fingers of dawn just reached out through the sky I woke your father and said, "It's time to go."

The birthing room was cold, sterile, silent, bright. It was an assault on my senses after the dark place I had come from. But I owned this experience and so we set about making it my den.

We turned the lights right down, the radio on, pushed the bed to one side and put blankets on the floor. Now I could birth.

They left me alone, didn't touch me, didn't measure me. I had told them before "Hands off." Your father made sure I didn't have to think of these things in this moment of intense birthing.

I walked.

I walked.

I dropped to the ground and roared with every contraction.

I pulled myself up again.

I walked....

There came a point where I clambered up onto the bed, got onto my knees and started screaming.

It was the most exquisite pain.

In between each contraction I laughed and smiled at your father. Partly to reassure him that I was fine even though I was screaming (I see now, the screaming made it fine, that's how I was dealing with the pain) b u t mostly because my body was making the most enormous amounts of endorphins. I was giddy and as high as I had ever been. It knocked my vision out and yet every moment is as clear as a bell.

I gripped the sides of the bed, tearing it.

I demanded ice be put to my lips.

I shouted "Come on baby, come on baby" to you to tell you the time had come.

Then it was over. I pushed once, twice, and you were in the world.

I was so tired I barely had the strength to turn and look at you. Your father held you as I moved my naked body around.

There you were. I held you on my chest. You didn't cry. I was naked, breathless and waiting for the afterbirth; I looked into your father's eyes with triumph.

I was the most powerful I have ever been; in that moment I had become the Goddess.

You nuzzled and crept until you found a nipple. You suckled.

You had come.

You were safe.

I love you.

HATHOR the COWGODDESS

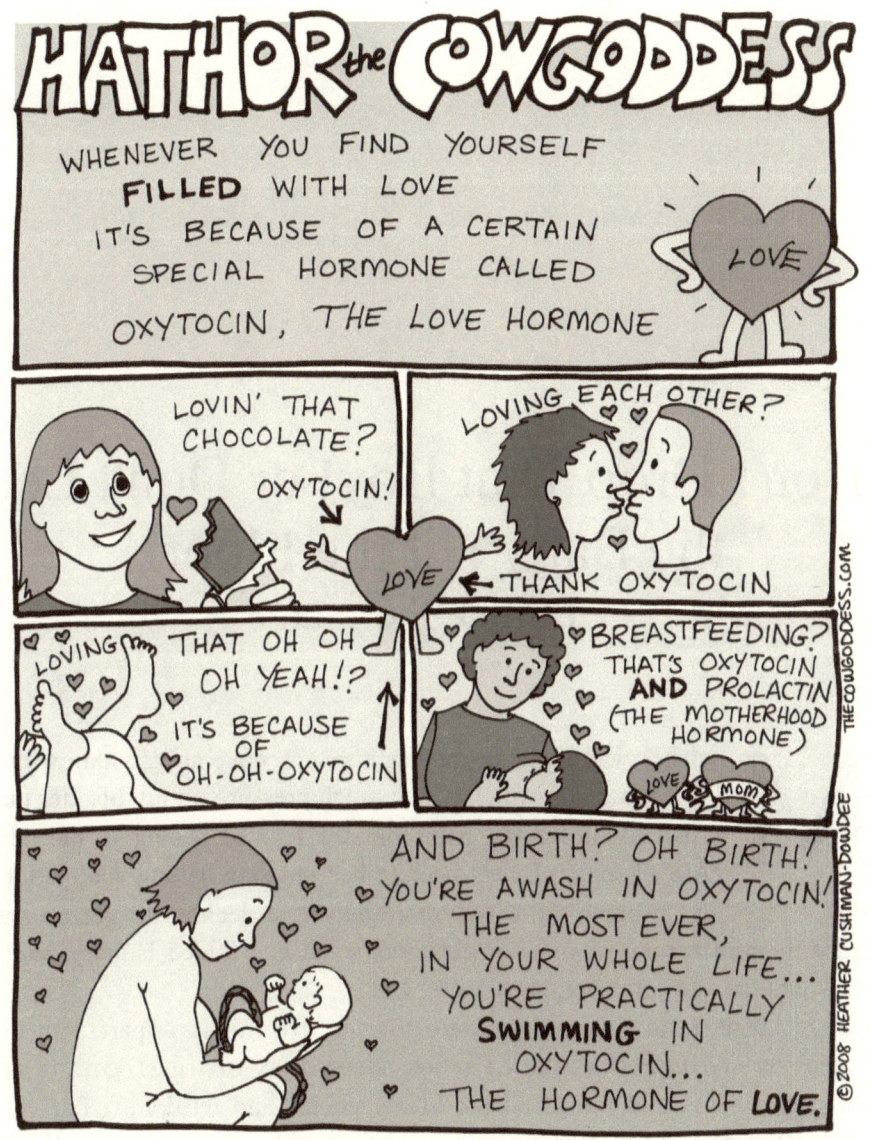

WHENEVER YOU FIND YOURSELF **FILLED** WITH LOVE IT'S BECAUSE OF A CERTAIN SPECIAL HORMONE CALLED OXYTOCIN, *THE LOVE HORMONE*

LOVE

LOVIN' THAT CHOCOLATE?

OXYTOCIN!

LOVE

LOVING EACH OTHER?

THANK OXYTOCIN

LOVING THAT OH OH OH YEAH!? IT'S BECAUSE OF OH-OH-OXYTOCIN

BREASTFEEDING? THAT'S OXYTOCIN **AND** PROLACTIN (THE MOTHERHOOD HORMONE)

LOVE   MOM

AND BIRTH? OH BIRTH! YOU'RE AWASH IN OXYTOCIN! THE MOST EVER, IN YOUR WHOLE LIFE... YOU'RE PRACTICALLY **SWIMMING** IN OXYTOCIN... THE HORMONE OF **LOVE.**

THECOWGODDESS.COM

©2008 HEATHER CUSHMAN-DOWDEE

31

Don't Drop That Boy! or Don't Let the Baby Hit the Floor!

Talitha Sherman

My labor was about as good as it gets. I woke at 2:55 a.m. with a big contraction which put so much pressure on my bladder that I had to run to the bathroom for fear of peeing in the bed. (Ain't I sexy?) I went back to bed but kept having contractions and became more and more awake. I decided to get up and putter till contractions stopped or got more intense. I folded laundry, had a snack and tea, did some computer work, etc.

About 5:30, contractions were four or five minutes apart. I lit the candles on my birth altar, started a fire, admired my offerings, got out my Blessingway box and reread all the lovely poems and wisdom. I felt very calm and didn't even want music to interfere with my inner voice. I just rocked forward over the birth ball with each contraction and went back to reading in between.

About 6:30 I felt I needed Dan's support. He soon saw that things were getting intense and wanted to call the midwife and Teri, who was going to watch the kids. I felt really uninhibited and didn't want anyone there yet, so he agreed to wait. I got in the shower till all the hot water was gone, stayed in the bathroom and got back in the shower when we had hot water again.

Being on my hands and knees during the contractions felt best. I sang "I Am Hollow Bamboo," a song that I learned at my Blessingway, during the contractions, which was an awesome way to focus and relax into them. Dan thought it was kinda weird, but in true Dan fashion, he was willing to support whatever worked for me. I'm sure he would have sung along if he'd known the words. The hot water was running out again, so Dan encouraged me to get out, worried about the cold raising my adrenaline levels and slowing labor. I did not want to stand up, and my contractions had just hit a new level of intensity, but I knew he was right.

I thought we should probably call people and wake the girls, but when I tried to stand, a huge tidal wave of pressure had me diving back onto my hands and knees and *push!* I felt a huge *pop!*

Dan says he saw water, bloody mucus (sorry, birth is messy you know) and vernix explode out of me.

I started screaming "Oh my god, the baby's coming!"

He said, "Okay, I'll call the midwife."

I screamed, "No, you don't understand! The baby's coming now!!"

So he went to call the midwife.

I was in a bit of a panic because I could feel the head coming but couldn't move or get up from my hands and knees in the bottom of the tub. I was scared that Dan would not be back to catch the baby.

He ran back in and turned off the water just as I pushed the head out. I could feel the burning and almost stopped pushing, but then I remembered that's how babies get out. Dan yelled something about the head being out, but I didn't care, I just knew I needed to push the rest out or it would never be over, so I pushed! I kept screaming, "Catch the baby!" Which woke the girls who got up and ran into the bathroom right behind Dan. Sadie said later she thought I was singing. Kira was first through the door and so was the only one to actually see the birth.

Dan announced, "It's a boy!"

All of the sudden, everyone was laughing and talking excitedly. Kira ran for the camera and Dan and I spent a couple of hysterical moments trying to figure out how to get me turned around in our never-seemed-so-small-before-tub without him dropping the baby or me getting tangled in the cord. We decided it would be the least mess and hassle to wait, deliver the placenta and then get me out of the tub. So I sat in the bottom getting to know my baby. The next half hour was so great. Just the six of us crammed into the bathroom. I think Hazel was the most excited. The girls took pictures and video and brought me towels and things.

Theo was amazing. He cried coming out, but calmed immediately and was nursing in no time.

And I am happy to report another big baby with no stitches!

Lucy's Birth
Amy Bell

My name is Amy Bell. I have two children. This is the story of Lucy my first born child. It feels important to acknowledge "Willow," the twelve-week-old fetus who left us two years before Lucy was born. Willow was my initiation. Lucy was my glorious journey into motherhood.

Lucy was twelve days past her due date when the gentle, almost ticklish twinges first occurred. Adam and I were brimming with excitement. The twinges started at 7 p.m. on May 15 (just like the dream I had my mother came to me and said, "Be ready for the fifteenth.") We put the mattress on the floor in the lounge room and tried to sleep. I got up every ten minutes with gentle twinges, they gradually started to build up to what was a strong contraction at 10 a.m. the next day. It was a really cold windy day, Adam had the potbelly stove going, and he kept running outside to get more wood and fixing the fence so that the dog wouldn't escape, but I don't remember him not being there. I started to enter a trancelike zone. A place of pain but happiness, excitement. I felt no fear. My body knew what to do, and I trusted. I moaned a low deep sound through the contractions and the pain would melt away to the edge of reality and I could 'see' the progress.

My friend dropped in to see how I was going at about 1:30 p.m. I remember feeling really tired and that the pain was too much, but she just said, "Keep going" or something like that and left. Adam and I, alone again, continued the labor. I would move from the toilet to the shower to the bean bag on the mattress covered with a shower curtain and blankets that I had set up in front of the potbelly stove.

At 5 p.m., on all fours, my body convulsed three times in a dry-wretch, and I knew that was "transition." After that, the pain that I had started to find unbearable vanished, and a new pain began. It was pleasurable. The baby's head entered the birth passage and began the journey out. Push by push, my body just delivered the child from me.

Then at 6:10 p.m., with a howl of glory, a cry of goddess-filled power, Lucy slid out into her dad's hands. The next moment I was holding her, shaking, lost in the bubble. I held her. She was still part of me, the cord between us still joining us. Over the next hour, we stood like that. Then the placenta decided it was time to leave. It felt soft and large leaving my body. I did a wee as the placenta emerged—and it stung! We put the placenta in a colander in a bowl and left the cord uncut until 10 p.m. that night. Adam cut the cold white cord and tied it with dental floss. The birth was over. We took Lucy into our bed and slept. (Except for Adam who stayed awake staring at Lucy all night.)

Adam's perspective: Amy knew it was starting to happen on Saturday and so I couldn't sleep because of anticipation of the unknown. It wasn't until Sunday night that the contractions became serious. We tried to sleep that first night because the contractions were not very strong or close together, but we didn't really sleep. The next day the labor seemed to really begin. Amy was coping well, mostly on the toilet, and in the shower, and leaning on the kitchen bench. Hot towels were a waste of time, instead Amy rubbed her forehead on my chest through the contractions (her forehead was raw by Lucy's arrival). In between all the contractions I was playing DJ and fixing the fence to keep the dog in. Why I didn't tie her up (the dog I mean) I don't know....I was also chopping firewood, it was freezing, and windy, and wet. It was a long day, I made myself food, but Amy didn't want any. A friend of ours came over to help, but Amy sent him away. Later in the day our Doula friend popped in, it was perfect timing, Amy had started to feel like she'd had enough, and the visit brought new energy and focus. After that, Amy really seemed to get into her head more, and it wasn't long before I caught my daughter. I think I said, "Oh, she's beautiful" or something. Lucy cried almost straight away, which was a relief because that meant she was breathing okay, but we had tried so hard to follow the "Fredrick Leboyer" way that I was hoping she would come out quietly. It was so fast, once her head was out I realized that the cord was around her neck. I attempted to push her back in and free the cord, but Amy gave one more push and Lucy slipped out at speed, I literally had to catch her. I handed her straight to Amy to feed, and we waited for the placenta. The excitement was very intense. After taking some photos in very low light without a flash, we got on our phones, too excited to care what a mobile call cost, or to wait our turns on the home phone; we rang our families simultaneously. That was the third night in a row without sleep, I lay awake buzzing, while Amy and Lucy slept, exhausted.

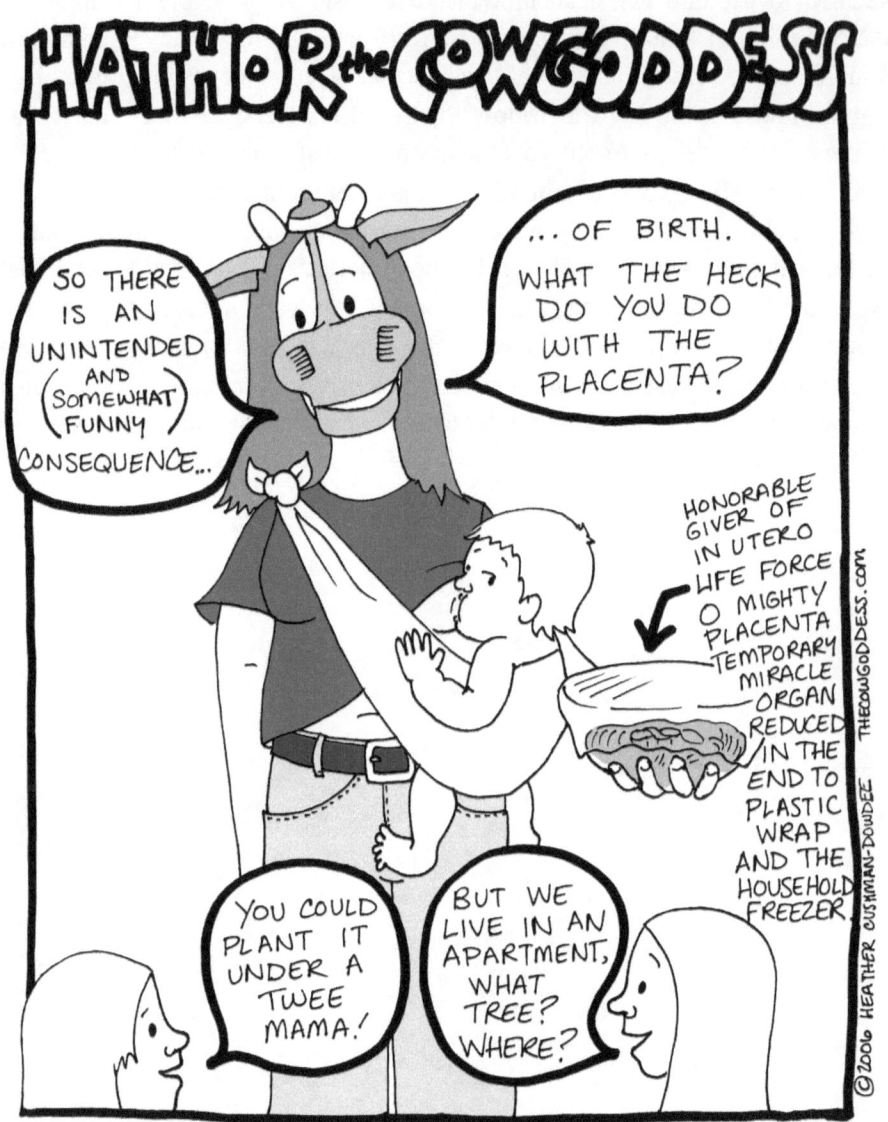

I Like to Move It, Move It!
Heather Farley

I was getting a little antsy about my baby coming. It was forty-two weeks and three days gestation from my last period and forty-three weeks gestation based on my ovulation date. I had been having regular Braxton Hicks contractions all week varying from three minutes apart to ten minutes apart.

Thursday, the 27th, Krysta, a friend from church came over and brought us split pea soup for dinner. We had just gotten up from a nap and had slept through dinner (that was my last "good" sleep). By the time we finished talking with her, I was trying to hide the fact that the contractions had just gotten stronger. It was 10:30 p.m. After we ate, I tried to lie down in our bath tub. At about midnight we went to bed. I struggled all night to sleep and eventually gave up at four in the morning. I remember looking over at my husband, McKay, thinking, "He shouldn't get to sleep if I can't!" So I woke him up.

Friday morning, I realized that we should probably blow up the birthing pool we borrowed. A friend of ours let us borrow a pump and McKay blew up the pool and filled it with hot water. During this time I was laboring on our birth ball and it felt pretty good. I tried some relaxation techniques that really helped control the contractions. In fact, McKay couldn't tell when I was having contractions. In my head, I was relaxed—I sent thoughts of "letting go" to my muscles. I was handling everything and was very calm.

Once the pool was filled I labored in it and McKay would make hot compresses out of washcloths and press them on my back for the pain and would boil water. I had made a list of birth affirmations; and he would read them aloud to me. He was doing the work of at least three people.

Most of Friday was just contraction after contraction of back labor. At some point I asked for a blessing from my husband, and I was told that I needed to be patient and that I would receive the inspiration on what to do next. That evening I started losing my mucous plug which was exciting because it meant progress was being made. Was it exciting! I think I was practically jumping up and down- and if I wasn't literally jumping, I definitely was inside. I continued losing my mucous plug up until Saturday morning. That night I pretty much didn't sleep and around five in the morning I was getting frustrated with the lack of progress. I was feeling like I didn't know what I was doing and the prospect of another full day of back labor was so overwhelming. It had been so long and so fruitless—or at least, I felt like there were no noticeable changes.

I had really hard back labor through the day. I threw up again sometime that afternoon, but we hid the clocks so I wouldn't be bothered by the time, so I don't know when. It was during this time that the labor was the toughest: It had been going on for a long time and I couldn't feel any progress.

The blessings I was given were my driving force. When I got frustrated, I would ask for another—I was reminded to have faith and patience; they helped me to pick myself back up and focus. One blessing in particular told me to remember all the women who had come before me and their strength and that I had that same strength. It was the words of the blessings that I would repeat in my head.

At some point, probably around 4 p.m., I realized that I didn't need McKay to apply pressure during the contractions. That meant either the baby was moving down or had moved down or that labor was going to be stalled. I was getting really tired of the back labor but was beginning to feel pushy. I wasn't sure how dilated I was so I didn't want to push too much, but I started vocalizing through contractions. I tried various positions—I had read that being on the toilet was helpful, but as soon as I tried, I knew it wouldn't be helpful to me. I also tried laboring on the birth ball, and in and out of the pool. I was up for anything.

Around 5:30 p.m., I started pushing with the contractions and could feel which contractions were productive and which weren't. I put my finger up my vagina and felt that the baby was about four inches back. I thought I felt the head, it was very smooth. "I feel the head!" I exclaimed. McKay and my friend, Jillynn, looked very happy. I felt reassured that this baby would come quickly. For the next while I would push with the contractions (and sometimes without contractions because I was so anxious to see my baby). I was finally making progress that I could measure, which gave me hope. I started ignoring the fact that I was supposed to wait for contractions and pushed whenever I got antsy. I discovered that pushing sort of induced a contraction: I would push without a contraction, but then my body would make a contraction and push with me. I was holding on to McKay's hands and leaning over the edge of the pool. I was telling myself, "I am not alone in this; many women have done this before. Their strength is my strength."

At some point in my pushing stage, the stereo played *I Like to Move It, Move It* by Reel 2 Real. I was doing lots of squats-up and down- and thought about how true it is that I like to "move it, move it." I told the baby that I wouldn't mind if it decided to "move it, move it" down the birth canal. Now when I look back on my birth, that's my theme song, though I didn't pay attention to which song was playing as she was born.

The next time I checked how far back the baby was, there was about an inch and a half to go! I was almost there!

McKay moved behind me into the water and I gripped Jillynn's hands. In the next few pushes I started feeling something crowning, but the ring of fire was not as strong as I expected. It was only a little bit of a sting. That's definitely not how I imagined the ring of fire at all! Ring of stinging, maybe, but no fire. I felt something hanging out of my vagina and put my hand down there and there was something really squishy. Weird. I thought my water had broken at some point in the pool and I had just not noticed. I stood up for McKay so he could see what it was. It was my bag of waters—I guess that's why I had never noticed it breaking.

I knew it was soon, so I gave a few more hard pushes and finally felt the ring of fire. (That's what I had been expecting!) The part that stung the most was up in front, I didn't feel any pain near my perineum. McKay saw the head coming, and I finished pushing it out. I knew at this point that there usually is a lull while the baby turns to get the shoulders through. I kept thinking McKay was pulling on the head and told him to stop. He said he wasn't. I felt the shoulders turn and I helped push them through. Two shoulders and an arm were pushed out, and then there was a slight pause before the rest of baby spilled out. The baby was still in the water sack until the feet came out, at which point it broke. McKay passed the baby to me between my legs and I brought it up out of the water for its first breath. I noticed she was a girl but didn't say anything yet. Jillynn and McKay started to help unwrap the cord which was around her arm. Boy, was she slippery! Then it was announced that we had a Margaret. We checked the time and it was 6:45. I had labored for forty-four hours.

When Margaret was born, she was very pink and started fussing and breathing right away. There was a good amount of vernix on her, which reassured me that she wasn't "overdue" and that everything was fine. There was a little stain of meconium on the top of her head, but that was it, and it was barely noticeable.

I started breastfeeding in the pool and then Jillynn suggested getting out of the pool and helped me out. I reclined on the couch, nursing our little Margaret. McKay gave me a blessing for the placenta to come quickly. I started noticing afterpains of my uterus clamping down as I was nursing (and, boy, were they intense)! About ten minutes after the birth, the placenta started coming out and was sitting in my vagina. I scooted towards the edge of the couch and it just fell out into a bowl with a lot of blood clots. Soon after, we grabbed our sterilized meat scissors and a piece of cotton yarn. The cord wasn't pulsing so I tied it off and McKay cut the cord. McKay examined the placenta and it was all there. I asked Jillynn at what point she thought I had hit transition. And she said, "A long time ago." I had shown signs that morning but none recently. Either that meant my second stage was really long or didn't really exist.

I did have some bleeding, and after some calls with local midwives, we decided to go to the hospital for stitches. I thought that maybe the tear was towards the front since that's where I felt the ring of fire, if it weren't for that, I don't think we would have gone. McKay had given me a blessing that I wouldn't hemorrhage or become unconscious and I trusted that. Someone (McKay? Jillynn?) snuck some cayenne tincture in my grape juice thinking it'd help any bleeding. All it did was give me an aversion to grape juice! Grape juice should NOT taste spicy!

Jillynn went to the hospital with me and I was stitched up—it did end up being only a perineal tear. Next time I'll be prepared with a mirror and a jug of water to wash away blood so I can diagnose my tears more easily. McKay brought Margaret up to the hospital for feeding and we left after a couple of hours (they wanted to monitor my bleeding in case of hemorrhage).

I had just given birth! I felt that I had made it through my rite of passage into motherhood. I was strong and had done something amazing. No more doubts, no more "what ifs," just pure, solid "I did it!" I went to sleep that night in my own bed with my husband and new daughter.

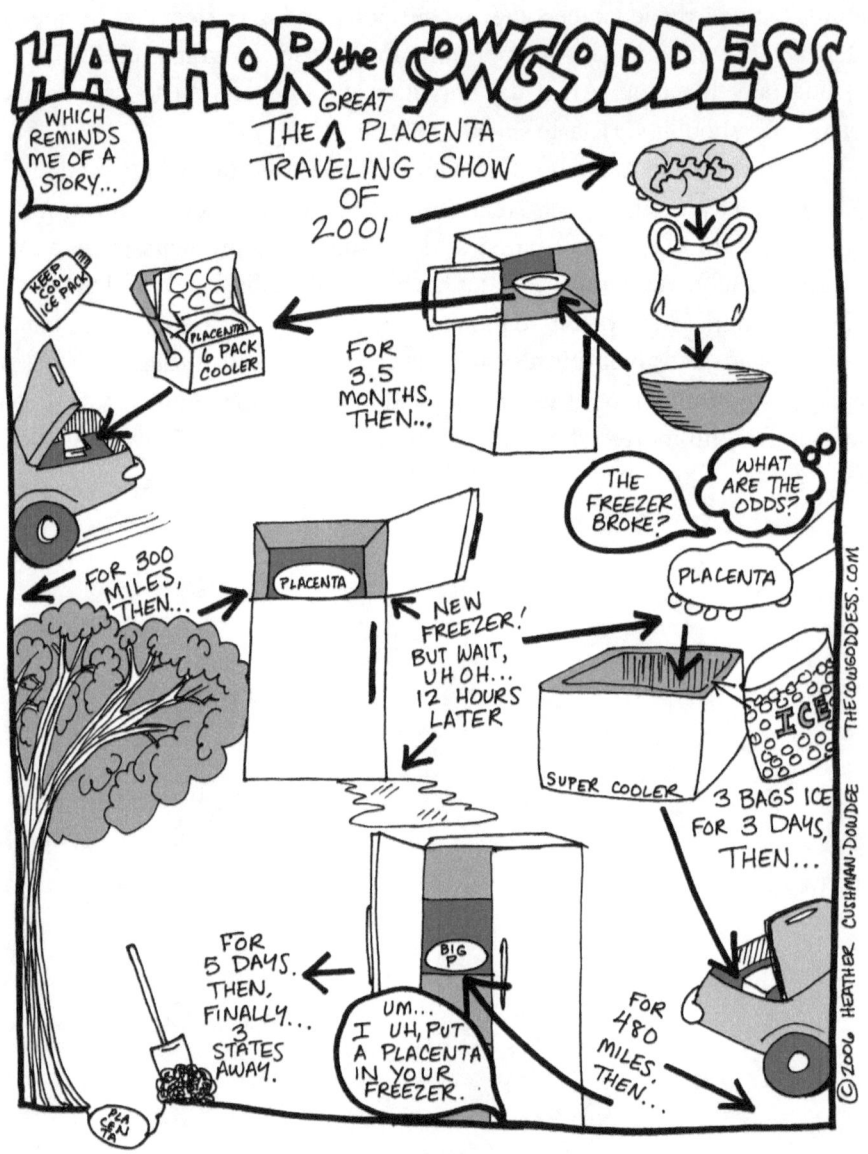

Just a Normal Day in the Life
Naomi Sand

After an hour or so, I told my husband Oscar and my daughter Samantha that it was time to get home from the farmer's market, early labor was starting to be just a little more than I was comfortable handling in public. At home, Oscar began doing some tidying-up task and then said he was just going to install the car-seat in our car. I guess I assumed he'd be right back. Samantha was asking a lot of questions. I tried lots of different positions and was pleased that I got to use the ball. Last time, I hadn't understood what it was for, but a friend explained how to use it, and it did feel quite nice. But only in a, "Cool, been-there-done-that" kind of moment; everything was happening so quickly that I was right on to the next thing.

Finally, Oscar returned and I found myself quite emotional, crying and saying to never leave for that long again. He had found that the perfect opportunity to clean the car. Men and their late nesting. Sheesh. Of course I had been in transition and the blessing is I had missed it! I needed to get into water and fast!

He got the bathtub filled and on the hot side as requested and then started working on filling the inflatable kiddy pool, which we'd set up in our bedroom. The reason the tub was hot was I'd just read that hot water slows labor and cooler water speeds it or allows it to progress at pace. But I didn't

45

really fit in that tub so I kept pouring water over my belly to try to keep things at bay and hollering for him to hurry up.

Finally, I couldn't wait any longer and I raced out of the tub and into the birth pool as it was being filled. Before I even hit the water, I was pushing. And crying out "No! Too fast, too fast baby, too fast!" But no, another strong contraction. How could this be possible? My first birth had taken hours, no, days of hard work. This was barely any labor at all and now I was pushing? Crazy!

I started to panic. And Oscar could see the fear in my eyes and reflected it back! For an awful moment, we were both on the verge of hysteria. And then my four-year-old channeled the collective birth wisdom and said, in a voice so calm and filled with authority, "Listen to your body, mommy," and we stopped. And we felt it. We felt the energy around us. We got calm. Everything after that moment was pure magic.

I reached down and felt my baby's head and felt smooth skin – my baby was still in the bag of waters! I could feel it! I could feel each little bit of progress and could see, ah, move a little here, yes, yes, a little this way, now like that. So easy!

And then a phrase came to mind: Ring of Fire. I guess I must have read that somewhere? I could visualize a rather large circle of absolute fire! It was awful! But so soon, it was done and my little baby was pushing so hard against my hand, I was pushing back with all my might to slow her down but still, she shot out like a bungee birth!

I wanted to let her take a minute to slowly rise to the surface of the water, knowing it was safe from all the videos I'd seen, but I just couldn't do it. I lifted her out and put her to my breast to nurse.

It was over and I'd done it! And I could do it again! Ahah! So that is why people had another child so soon after their first child. After a birth like that, I could do anything. The magic was still all around us. The channels to the other world were wide open. The air was sparkly all around us. It was not how I'd pictured it, but it was amazing and I was amazing and we were all amazing! And again, that sense of being part of something so, so much bigger than just myself and our little lives.

And this perfect little baby! There she was! So warm and slippery and wet and real and heavy! And seriously cute!

But now the water was so deep that I could not really keep her face out of the water. So we decided to get out of the pool. Only I hadn't birthed the placenta yet and the cord was so short. Oscar held my little lion cub (who we were already calling by her name because I was right; she was a girl, and I was the only one who was right) and I stepped very awkwardly out.

In hindsight, that must have been when it happened. There was very little blood in the pool but the midwife, who we invited to come right after I got out, discovered that the towels on the bed were so, so heavy with blood. I don't know how this next bit happens but it is a full five hours of the midwife being with us, sweetly being part of the energy, gently trying to convince me to either pee so the placenta will come out or let her cut the cord. Oh, and she wanted to know would I please, please stop that annoying habit of fainting while she was talking to me?

I remember being flat on my back on the floor, unable to get up, but the baby barely able to nurse because of that short cord, me still naked and having hot and cold flashes, everyone rushing to crank the air conditioning, no wait, turn on the heat!

My sweet husband and daughter crawl into bed with my new little lion cub. Although I miss her, I am so glad we had a home birth and she is in her own bed with her own family. Such a sweet image. It is nearly midnight and they finally get some much-needed rest.

My midwife convinces me to muster enough strength to do some kind of crazy back slide to the bathroom and into the tub. Now I'm ready to fully focus on me. I had been trying homeopathic and other remedies for the last 4 hours to either get the placenta out or pee; she felt that if I peed, the placenta would be freed up. She is certain I will be able to pee in the tub and she is right! I do manage to pee finally, but no placenta. So I reach down and wouldn't you know it – the darned thing was hanging at the back door all that time. Remember how I'd reached down and felt smoothness instead of hair? Well, that was the bag of waters but she was not born in it; it had torn right there so it must have been blocking the placenta. My midwife had me cough and, "Poof" out came the placenta, which I'd effectively already birthed and it was just needing that last helping push to come out.

So the happy ending is that I did rebuild my blood over the next weeks and months using alfalfa pills and organic electrolyte drinks. Friends and acquaintances were so movingly amazing, dropping food by at least daily and sometimes twice daily for an entire month. We needed the help very much and I am so grateful for what we received and for this perfect birth!

My Journey to VBAC
Lynn Grabowski

At 5:20 a.m., on March 28th 2004, I woke up because I just couldn't get comfortable. I used the bathroom and tried to get back to bed but couldn't get comfy, so I got up and got online for a while. I started feeling regular contractions about fifteen minutes apart. I told my husband and said he could go back to sleep to which he replied, "Yeah, right." He ran to the store and picked up some milk and a few other things since he wouldn't get the chance later.

I sat on my birth ball and sniffed a lavender aromatherapy pillow. I began to pace around the house, as contractions got stronger and closer together. I tried to eat but felt a little queasy so I drank some Gatorade instead. I'd made up some of my own labor-ade ice cubes and sucked on those. I took a shower and when the hot water died on me all too soon I decided to get into the hot tub. The contractions picked up stronger and faster once in the tub, and I started feeling pushy. But, after twenty minutes of pushing and it just not feeling right, I decided to get out of the tub. I put some chux pads down on my bed and lay on my left side for a while as I'd read that was supposed to slow things down but it didn't help much. I also started having some back labor at that point and needed my husband to provide lots of counter-pressure on my lower back to help. I sat on the birth ball, showered again, and moved around a lot, but the contractions started coming right on top of each other, so I got back in the tub. We sat in there a long time with my husband pressing on my back. My son helped some, cheering me on and holding my hand on occasion. He mostly stayed inside watching movies. I used lots of vocalizing and breathing techniques to help as well.

Around 2 p.m. I started feeling pushy again and this time it felt *so* good to push. I could tell I had hit transition because I started feeling like I couldn't do it and burst into tears for what seemed like no real reason. I was tired and wanted desperately to just sit and put my knees together, but I could feel his head right in my pelvis and it just hurt to lean back. If I had one thing to do differently I would have taken prenatal yoga to stretch and strengthen my thigh muscles, I think it would have helped immensely! After I started pushing I stayed on all fours with my husband pressing my lower back with each contraction. Boy, were his arms tired the next day!

I eventually started to feel the head descend with each push. The contractions still hurt as they rose, but when I pushed with them it just felt amazing! My husband really coached me and let me know he could feel the baby descending. At one point, he accidentally poked the head and I felt my son move inside me it was so strange! I hadn't experienced any of this in my first labor.

When the head began to emerge my husband said he felt something squishy, and I reached down and felt something soft and pulsing and momentarily thought it was the cord. I tried not to panic and looking back on it I knew deep down nothing was wrong, but I had my husband call 911 just in case. (In retrospect even if it had been the cord, if it were still pulsing then it was still moving oxygen to the baby anyhow!) As he called I got up in a half squat, one knee up, one kneeling, and I started to push like crazy knowing if the cord was there I had to get him out *now*. As he started to emerge more I realized it was just where the bones in the head fold up during delivery and nothing was wrong. I still pushed like crazy since my husband was still on the phone, and he gave the dispatcher the play by play as if it were a baseball game. "The head is crowning, wait it's out, wait there's the body! It's out, the baby is crying, and fine!!" I felt the head pop out and the body shot out into the water on the next contraction. He was born posterior-face up! I pulled him up out of the water and cried "I did it, we have a baby!" the 911 dispatcher asked, "So, is it a boy, or a girl?" we hadn't even thought to look yet! We looked and told him it was a boy, he congratulated us, asked if we still needed them and we said no, thanks so much, and got off the phone.

We went inside to warm up the baby. (I imagine at this point I might have shocked some neighbors as I'd just given birth naked on my porch but no one has said anything yet!) The cord was very short and I had to waddle with him at my belly button level. It couldn't have been much more than a foot long. My husband laid him on the bed and covered him with warm towels from the dryer. He was taking a long time for his limbs to pink up so we suctioned him a little and worked on warming him up. I couldn't nurse with the cord so short, so we waited for it to stop pulsing and turn white and we cut it. I had wanted to wait for the placenta initially but it was just too awkward to care for him.

I took some angelica tincture to help ease the placenta and my husband dried off the baby and got him dressed. I tried to squat over a bowl to deliver the placenta but I was *so* tired I just couldn't do it. A few more contractions came on so I knew it would probably come out soon. I went and sat on the toilet and nursed my newborn son; the placenta fell out a few minutes later. I scooped it out and put it in the bowl I'd originally planned to use, passed my son to my husband and got in the shower to clean up. Even with all that hard fast pushing I only had a tiny tear that I didn't even notice till about a week later after it had all but healed up. My husband weighed the baby while I was showering; he weighed 8 pounds 6 ounces. My first son had been 6 pounds 11 ounces. It always amazes me how VBAC babies are so much bigger!!

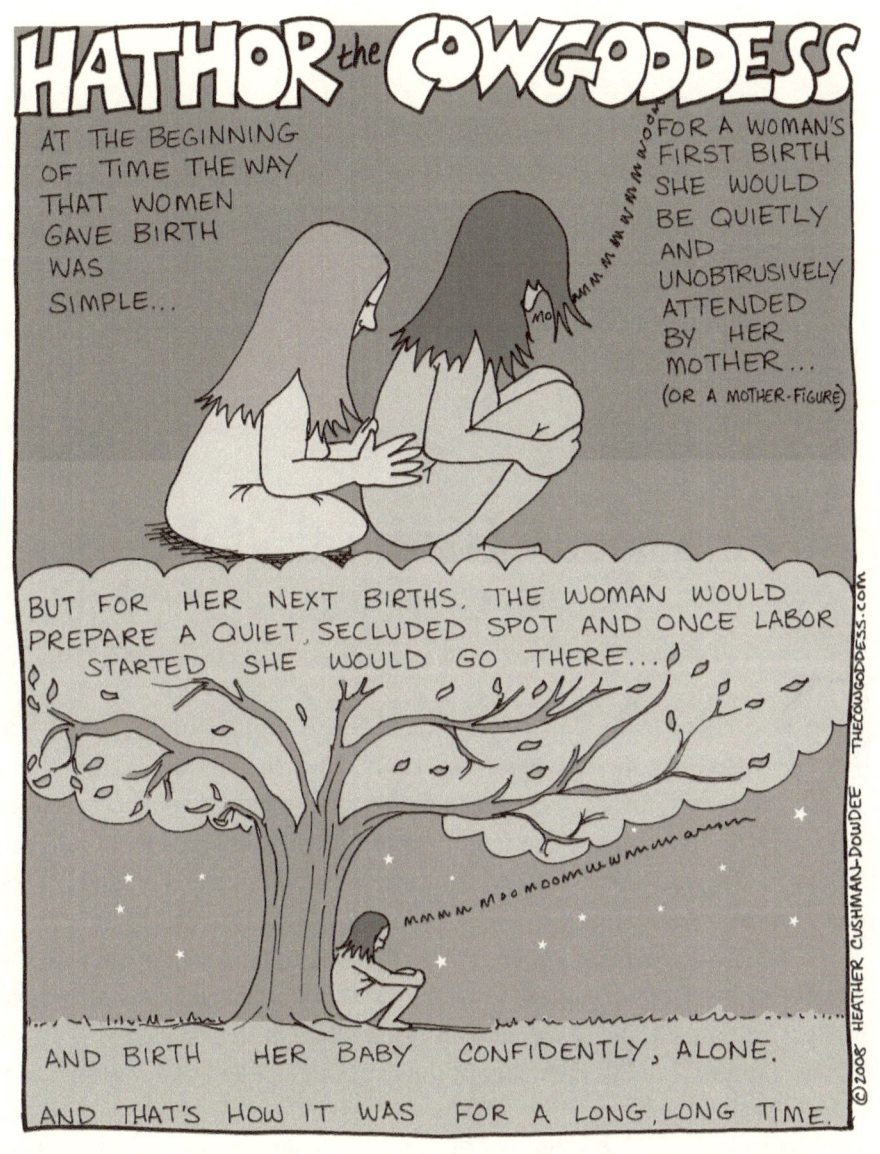

The Speedy Birth of Nicholas
Lynn Grabowski

December 29th, I woke up around 3 a.m. to use the bathroom like usual. I noticed when I lay back down that I was having slight contractions. At this point I didn't think much of them. They were regular, maybe five minutes apart, and almost pleasant in sensation. I decided to stay in bed a while since I'd had contractions much like this on and off for about the past week.

4 a.m. I woke up again to use the bathroom and notice that the contractions were coming closer together and that I felt more comfortable while sitting on the toilet. I stayed there for a while, trying to decide whether this was it or not. I didn't have any of the usual signs I had with my first two so I went back to bed.

4:40 a.m. All of a sudden the pleasant contractions gave way to a very hard sharp contraction that really got my attention. I definitely couldn't stay in bed any longer. I got up again and went to get a glass of water. The hard strong contractions continued to come and I decided it was time to wake up my husband. He went to fill the pool only to find the hose connections he was planning to use (on the washing machine) were rusted tight and all of his tools were 45 minutes away with his airplane. He ran to the store to get a pair of pliers and I got into the bathtub. I wasn't able to get the bath water high enough to be really useful and the floor of the tub was so hard that it was uncomfortable on my hips. It was better than nothing however and as a bonus my bathtub has a strong handicap bar in it that I was able to pull on during the contractions. When my husband got home he started working on getting the pool filled. I began to moan through the pains as they took more of my attention. I think this got his attention as well. My last two labors had at least five hours of the easy stuff and this was coming on fast. I got into the pool the second it began to fill so I could help gauge the water temp, and get the benefit as soon as possible. The water only got about a third of the way full when the hot ran out so I sat in there and figured we could add more later if needed. Shortly after this the contractions began to come in waves. I was thankful that I got a small twenty-second or so break between them but each one came back with the strength of a runaway train. I felt like I was pulled in every direction with each one. I've never experienced anything so intense. Hubby provided some counter-pressure on my lower back, which helped a little at first and later became more of just something else to focus on. I tried to breathe through them when possible, but things got faster and faster.

6:25ish a.m. Suddenly, I felt an urge to push. I had a moment of doubt because I'd had an early urge to push with my last labor that just turned out to be my water about to break. I pushed slightly and sure enough my water did break with that one. I had enough wherewithal to briefly ask my husband if the water was clear and get his confirmation before I was hit with a rush of hormones. I suddenly broke into sobbing tears that I couldn't really explain. The urge to push didn't go away. I tried to breathe through the next two pushes still doubting them, and then on the third, my body took over and the baby's head slid instantly to crowning. Again I tried to breathe hoping not to tear. The burning was intense. I wasn't able to hold off and his head was out on the next contraction. At this point I had a slightly longer break between contractions and yelled to my husband to support the head. I also remember saying to just pull him out already, but I'm glad he didn't hear that part! My husband was surprised because he hadn't even realized the head was out until I'd said something. It all happened so quickly. On the very next contraction his body slid out and into my husband's hands. I was so shocked momentarily because I hadn't expected it all so fast. I sat and he handed me the baby who immediately let out a wail and pinked up beautifully. I sat in the pool a moment, close to one of the pool heaters to

53

keep baby and me warm and waited for the cord to stop pulsing. Once it did, hubby cut and tied it and I handed him the baby to go show the boys.

6:31a.m. I waited for the placenta which delivered easily. I examined it and put it in a bowl for the meanwhile. The boys came running in excited. My three-year-old said to me, "Mom look the baby is here!" as if I had missed it!

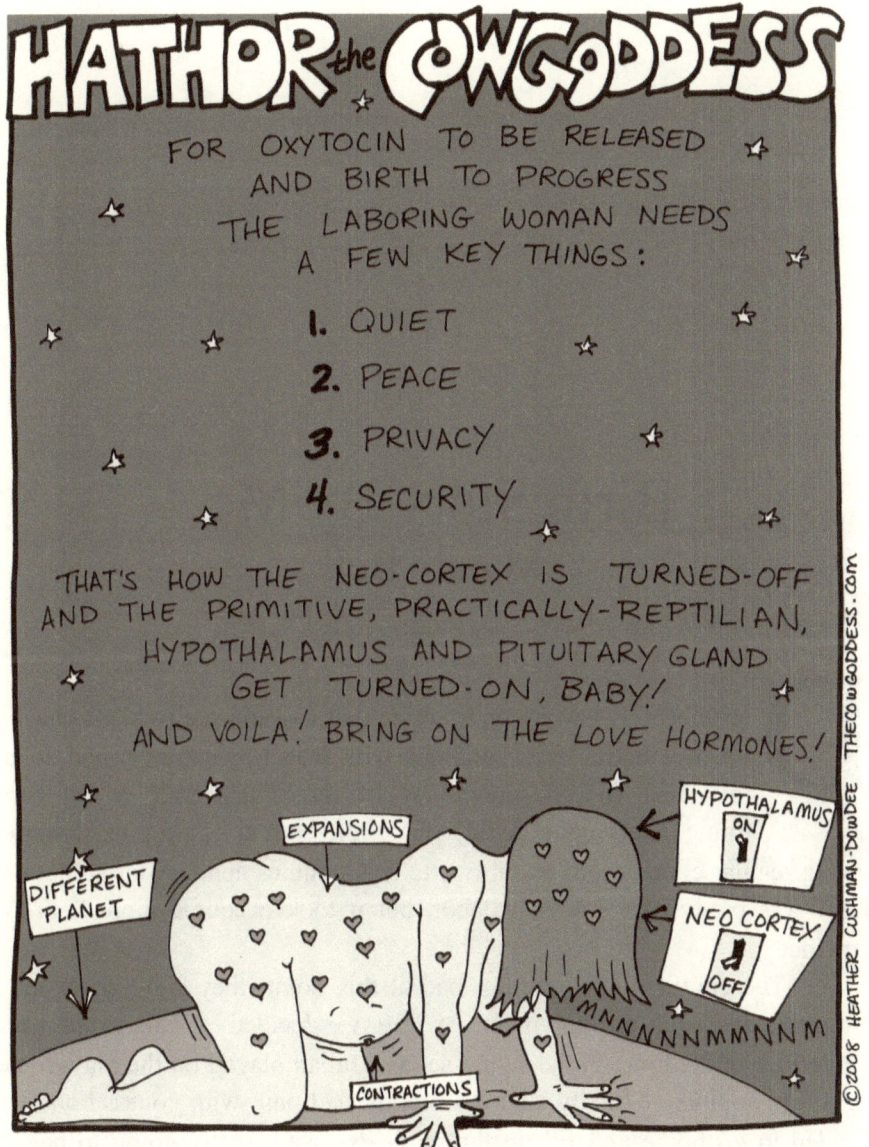

HATHOR the COWGODDESS

FOR OXYTOCIN TO BE RELEASED
AND BIRTH TO PROGRESS
THE LABORING WOMAN NEEDS
A FEW KEY THINGS:

1. QUIET
2. PEACE
3. PRIVACY
4. SECURITY

THAT'S HOW THE NEO-CORTEX IS TURNED-OFF
AND THE PRIMITIVE, PRACTICALLY-REPTILIAN,
HYPOTHALAMUS AND PITUITARY GLAND
GET TURNED-ON, BABY!
AND VOILA! BRING ON THE LOVE HORMONES!

EXPANSIONS

DIFFERENT PLANET

HYPOTHALAMUS
ON

NEO CORTEX
OFF

MNNNNNMMNNM

CONTRACTIONS

©2008 HEATHER CUSHMAN-DOWDEE THECOWGODDESS.com

Birth Story By Me,
Mandy Bell

Dec\ecember 21, I woke up thinking that I would really like to have a Solstice baby. I ate breakfast with Rob (my partner) and Julian (my first son, a month shy of three) and took a hot bath. Immediately upon getting out of the bath at 12:45 p.m., I started having regular contractions about two to five minutes apart. After an hour of this I was pretty sure I was in labor, but it took a couple more hours to convince me.

The contractions were not bad at this point; they were short and I could talk and walk through them. At 2:30, we decided to walk to the park, where Rob pushed me on the swing-set and Julian played on the playground for a few minutes. I finally started to really feel pain with contractions and decided to go home and fill up the pool—we were really going to have a baby!

At home, we had all kinds of issues filling the pool up, and Robert made about thirty trips up and down the stairs with pots of boiling water because the hot tap water kept running out so quickly. Once the water was ninety degrees and about halfway full, around 4 p.m., I got in and stayed in until after the birth. The two times I got out to go to the bathroom were excruciating; the contractions were totally unbearable out of the water.

The contractions stayed at about every three minutes from very early in labor until Luka's birth—they got longer and stronger, but not closer together. I was really starting to lose control at this point, my relaxation techniques were barely keeping me going. I kept saying, "I can't do this," which I continued to repeat until I started pushing. I checked my cervix and saw little progress around 6 p.m. I couldn't believe that the past five hours had done nothing for me and was really disappointed (this is why people advise against cervical checks in labor, of course).

After 6:30, I started to make progress and dilated pretty quickly. The contractions were long and very painful, I shifted positions every which way to try to get comfortable during them, and it didn't work. The best position was hands and knees or elbows and knees, but my arms were so shaky by the end of a contraction my face would be almost in the water. My mom showed up at seven-something and she and Rob sat and talked with me during the two minutes of contraction-free time.

Around 8:15 or so I checked myself and found myself complete, but waited a couple of contractions until I felt the urge to push. I pushed for four or five contractions, about ten minutes total. The first one I wasn't sure if I was pushing or not, but after the second I said, "I'm pushing!" and they said, "We know." After the third contraction his head was *right* there about to be born and I said, "Oh my god, there's a person in me!" It felt so strange. The next contraction brought his head most of the way out, and I paused to stretch with him. After his head, it seemed to me like a long time before his body came out but Rob and my mom said it was immediate. I must have been in some weird time warp. He was born around 8:30 p.m. (we didn't think to check the time for several minutes, oops)! I pushed his head out on hands and knees, and caught his body kneeling, pulling him up to me. I was so ecstatic and amazed that I didn't think to do anything but throw a warm towel over him and stare. It took quite a while before I thought to check between his legs, and when I did I said, "Hi baby boy! Hi Luka!" He was covered from head-to-toe in thick vernix, which is odd at thirty-nine plus weeks. I rubbed it in with the wet towel I had over him.

After a couple of minutes of me staring at him lying there, I thought he wasn't breathing. His eyes were closed and he was still. I rubbed his back, and listened closely, only to realize he was asleep! After a few minutes he woke up and looked around suspiciously.

I held him on my chest in the tub for about forty-five minutes waiting for the placenta, until the water started to feel chilly and I decided to get out. I handed Luka to Rob, still attached to me by a fairly short umbilical cord (Rob had to hold him at waist-level), got out of the pool, and birthed the placenta into a bowl. Rob grabbed the cord tape and we tied and cut Luka's cord, which at that point was totally white and cold. I left Luka with Rob and went into the bathroom to shower—Luka got weighed and I was shocked to hear he weighed 9 pounds I had expected a big baby, but he looks so small!

I can't believe I did it! It was soooo hard and definitely painful, but I am so happy to have gotten my "sweet little squishy face" out of it.

As Mother Nature Intended
Lauren Jackson

The baby was "due" on October 10. I had been having mild contractions on the evening of October 9, starting at about 7 p.m. A couple of them were a little intense; there was no pain or anything, but I had a *lot* of pelvic and rectal pressure. My husband Roger and I had sex late that night to try to move things along a bit. I had some contractions overnight, they woke me up maybe three times, but again, they were mild so I was able to drift back to sleep easily. I got woken up by one at about 5:30 a.m. that was pretty intense. I got up to go to the bathroom a few minutes later and had lots of blood-tinged mucous. Roger woke up to go to work and I told him that he wouldn't be going in today, that the baby was coming. He snoozed for a while, resting up for the big event and snuggling with Lucas, our two-year-old son, who was still sleeping in our family bed.

At one point, I threw-up until there was nothing left. The contractions were already about five to six minutes apart and were intense. I dozed off between contractions; I was thankful for the rest.

Mom arrived a short time later to look after Lucas. My best-friend Barbara helped Roger set up the pool and all the necessities from my "to-do list," while I labored in the tub for a little while longer. Then Barbara helped me run to the pool before another contraction hit.

It felt so good to be in there; I can't even imagine how women go through this without being immersed in water. It made it so much more bearable.

After a little while, Roger got in with me and sat behind me and massaged and applied pressure to my lower back during each contraction. Barbara stayed outside the pool at my head, stroking my hands and arms and talking me through them.

It's amazing how my mind kept working and continued to be aware of everything even in the middle of contractions. I even kept up with the time and made sure that the moms made Lucas' lunch on time. I watched HGTV between contractions, to help me focus and regroup. Labor seemed to go on forever, but every time I looked at the clock, only fifteen minutes had passed. I remember thinking during one particularly intense contraction that I couldn't do this anymore, but then when it let go, I felt like "of *course* I can do this!" I remembered that women have been birthing for eons and eons without assistance, and I reminded myself just to take it one contraction at a time and not think about anything other than the present moment. I trusted my body and knew it would take care of things on its own.

The contractions very quickly got to two to three minutes apart. A couple of times I had three right on top of each other; they didn't even go all the way down before another one started. I knew I was getting close at this point, and I was *so* ready for it to be over.

I laid on my side for a long time, propped up on my elbow, with my head against the side of the pool. After a while, that didn't feel like the right position to be in anymore, so I moved up to my knees, draping my arms over the side of the pool. During the peak of the contractions, my body started bearing down, pushing. I thought to myself that it seemed awfully soon for this to be happening, but I went with it and just let it happen. It's not like I could have stopped it anyway.

But, oh my God, bearing down felt so good. All the pain of the contractions just stopped completely.

Roger got out of the pool to go to the bathroom and to move around a little bit, and I decided to check my cervix, the first out of only two times anyone did so. It felt like this huge cavernous opening; it was amazing. I felt as though if I gazed through it, I could see the vast expanse of the universe on the other end. After a few more pushes, I reached up and checked again, and I felt the amniotic sac poking down through the opening. I mentioned this to Barbara and told her it would be breaking soon. It did on the next contraction, as my body bore down. It made an audible pop that Barbara even heard through the water and she felt the popping sensation radiate through my body from where her hands were on my shoulders.

Roger came back a few minutes later, and I told him it wouldn't be much longer. He got back into the pool with me, sitting behind me to apply counter-pressure and massage my lower back.

A few contractions later, I reached up to check the baby's progress, with the tip of my two fingers, I could feel the top of his head at the mouth of the cervix.

The bearing-down contractions continued for a while, and very soon, I felt the baby moving down the birth canal. I stayed on my knees with my arms draped over the side of the pool. When bearing down during one contraction, I felt a huge crack in my pelvic region and everyone in the room heard a tremendous "pop" noise. That was my tailbone dislocating as the baby's head moved past it. It wasn't painful until much later. We all just wondered what it was, but I was pretty sure it was my tailbone because I had read somewhere that it could dislocate during the pushing stage.

My body started pushing really hard, and his head started crowning very quickly. I yelled out to my mother-in-law that if my mom and Luke wanted to see the birth, they'd better get in here *now*, so she ran to the bedroom to get them. They all came back in the room, and my body kept pushing, and the baby's head was halfway through. Lucas and Mom stood beside the pool looking down at me, Lucas was staring intently. Roger was behind me in the pool; I laid back into his arms and pushed the head the rest of the way out. What a relief! I didn't feel any "ring of fire" that people describe, which I attribute to being in the water. I sat and rested for a few seconds, waiting for the next contraction. I felt his body turning, and I said, "He's turning!" A contraction hit right then, and on October 10 at 2:02 p.m., I pushed Connor Vance out into the water, into my own hands. The time between when his head came out and his body passed through was only a few seconds, and I think I pushed for a little over an hour. He landed in my hands, but then slipped right through them and into Barbara's hands where she had them underneath mine just in case that happened. He was so slippery! Barbara and I pulled him up out of the water together and I laid him across my arm so all the fluid could drain from his mouth and lungs.

Connor started crying almost immediately, and, boy, did he have a set of lungs! Roger and I laid him down on my chest together, and Roger wrapped his arms around us. We covered Connor and I up with a big bath towel, I cuddled him close to get him warm, and he calmed down a bit. A few minutes later, I felt like I really needed to get out of the pool, and I wanted to birth the placenta in the bathtub. Barbara and Roger walked me to the bathroom while I carried the baby. I stepped into the tub (which was still full of water from that morning), knelt down, grunted once and the placenta came out into the water. It was 2:13 p.m., eleven minutes after Connor was born.

Barbara put the placenta into the metal bowl I provided and examined it thoroughly as I had instructed (it was perfectly intact) and then she and Roger helped me dry off and move to the bed.

Roger tied off and cut the umbilical cord maybe an hour and a half or two hours after Connor was born, and he was finally a whole separate being. I eventually got back into the bathtub, still holding Connor because he wouldn't let me put him down, so I could take a sitz bath with herbs to help soothe the "skid mark" he left on his way out (I didn't tear, it was more like a scrape.)

After he pooped several times and nursed a lot, we finally got around to weighing him that evening. He was 7 pounds 6 ounces.

Birth Story
Jess Urwin

I woke Wednesday, March 16, with contractions. I lay in bed through a few but, didn't pay any attention to how long or far apart they were. To be honest I was trying to fall back to sleep. At 7 a.m. I needed to go to the bathroom so I got up and realized that, "Today is probably the day." I started filling the tub and posted to my groups that I had changed my mind about being pregnant forever. My body also took care of some house cleaning at this point.

When Tony got home it was hard for him to split his attention between me and the kids so he got pretty stressed, but he was great about getting things for me and generally setting up things. I lost all track of time. The contractions were intense but bearable and I got out of the tub several times to pee. Going pee was a very precise operation. I absolutely cannot stand to have a contraction on the toilet so I had to wait until I was just getting over a contraction then jump (Jump? I was nine months pregnant and in labor, "Jump!" Ha, snort.) out and run to the toilet and hope that I was done and off before the next one started. Several times Tony had to rescue me from the toilet.

Dria was so great, she would hold my hand during contractions and she felt that it was her personal duty to get me anything I asked for. I was alternating between kneeling and squatting, facing sideways in the tub. Between contractions I would lay my head on the side of the tub and doze. At this point my legs were really cramping up from being bent for so long so I tried side-lying in the tub and that was not a great position, so I went back to my squatting and kneeling.

For some reason during this labor I was really thinking about pooping during pushing, it was something I was wasting a lot of energy on. I really did not want to poop in the tub so I kept getting out and trying to go on the toilet but nothing was happening. I had Tony get me a chux pad to squat on and I tried pushing there so if I pooped it wouldn't be in the water, to no avail. And contractions on land were much worse than in the water so I finally decided I would just deal with whatever happened.

After I got back in the water, I checked my cervix to see what was going on. I could only feel one side of my cervix and the bag of waters was bulging at the cervix, I could also feel the baby's head through the bag. I remembered the first time I felt during Kaia's birth, her head was barely one knuckle in and I felt a bit discouraged that it was all the way up by my cervix.

I tried pushing a bit and all of a sudden I no longer had a choice about pushing. I was in a really funny position, my legs would no longer hold me in a squat so I was kind of kneeling but leaning off to one side. I was worried about getting too high because I didn't want the baby's head to be out of the water at any point and then I would have to get out of the water to finish delivering him. Tony said something to me about not banging his head on the bottom of the tub. So we each had our own worries.

Tony kept telling me to slow down so I wouldn't tear and I just didn't have any choice. I was rubbing the baby's head through it all, which really helped me to concentrate and ride through the contractions. My body was doing it all and I had the irresistible urge to push.

Finally my water broke and I could feel his head at my perineum, I also felt the ring of fire, ouch. Then his head was born and I felt his face and could feel these incredibly chubby cheeks and then I felt him turn to face my right thigh and then the rest of him slid out. I pulled him to my chest and leaned back on the end of the tub.

We called Tristan over to check the sex; he said, "It's a boy!" Then I moved the cord out of the way and asked him if he was sure and he just said,

"Oh," in a disappointed tone and walked out of the room. Poor Tristan, he so wanted a brother since he already had two sisters.

Tony announced that it was 11:13. Shortly after, I got into a squat and pushed and out came the placenta and I sort of pulled the bits of membrane out after it. We were just sure through the whole pregnancy that the baby was a boy, so we had no name for this little girl baby.

Tony went and boiled the scissors to cut the cord. I was not in a hurry to cut the cord, but Tony was. He asked me how short to cut the cord and I told him that it didn't matter to just cut it so he cut it about six inches from the baby. Then Tony took the baby and wiped her off while I had a quick shower and kind of cleaned out the tub. Then I took our newest baby back and went to relax in the living room.

It wasn't until the next morning that we came up with a name for this surprise baby girl. Tony suggested Nahlia. So Nahlia Roe she is. We didn't weigh or measure her that first day, but on Thursday we took her to the pediatrician and she was 8 pounds 13 ounces, and 20.5 inches long. She was one of my smaller babies.

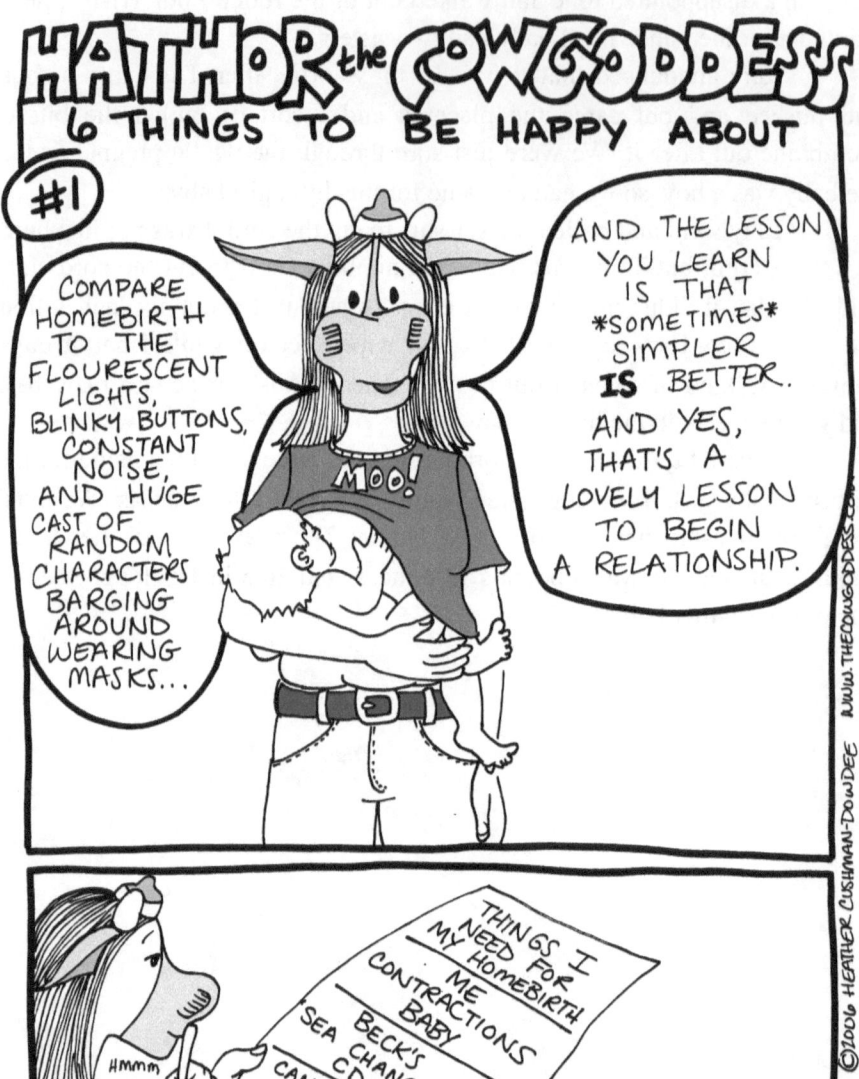

Rowan's Birth Story
Heather Hawkes

At 11 p.m. every one of the kids is asleep (even our night owls). Mike is pooped from getting up so early (5:30 a.m.) and I tell him to just get some sleep (as he needs to be functional tomorrow with the kids) and I will wake him up if I need him. I draw myself a nice hot bath and soak and have wonderful contractions, noting to myself that the stronger they get the more my back is starting to hurt. Around 2 a.m. I give my friend a call. She is there by 2:45 or so. Time for me seems to be going by so fast. The contractions are now feeling very strong. I am not tired, I feel great...but my back is really starting to hurt a lot when I have a contraction.

I wake Mike up and tell him Alica and I are going for a walk and we will be back soon. It is a very short walk as I have to pee right away. But it is a good walk and I have six or so contractions while we are walking. After going to the bathroom I draw another bath. Alica and Mike join me in the bathroom and we chat. Of course by now all the noise has woken up Sis who comes in to use the bathroom and then can't get back to sleep. At 4:30 a.m., I am feeling like I am in transition. The contractions are so overwhelming and by now my back is just screaming. I want to have a water birth, but I cannot get into a position that feels good to my back. So out of the tub and into the bed I go. Alica puts some good counter-pressure on my back. Mike goes and

67

gets Sis and Logan who come in and start giggling at all the noises I am making...which is exactly what I need to sort of snap me back to earth and focus. I start feeling "pushy" and my lovely husband places a nice warm compress on my perineum. *One huge push* and out pops Rowan in all his big beautiful glory. He is so calm and quiet, he goes right to my chest and we rub him a little as he is bluish on his fingers and toes. He has a great big wail and pinks up. He nurses right away.

After a bit the placenta finally comes out while I am on the toilet trying to pee. Totally grosses Sis out.

It was a very empowering experience, being totally in control of my own birth. Not having fear, not giving up my power. Having who I wanted there and doing what felt right to me.

Yes, parts were intense, but it was good. It was very good. It was a beautiful way to end my baby-making years.

The Epic Birth of Eli
Jen Holland

I woke up Friday morning to what seemed like some regular contractions, so I decided to time them for a while to appease my curiosity. I had four clockwork contractions, ten minutes apart, the first regularity to this labour so far! I told Nick and the kids that today was going to be our day.

We stuck around the house and while my contractions continued and increased in intensity, they were still far apart and pretty short. I considered my options for spurring the labour on—spicy food? sex? long walk?—and decided to just chill and let it happen. At some point in the afternoon, though, I started to feel like a watched pot. I began to feel a little bit disheartened (I'm going to be in labour forevvvvver!) and texted a good friend that maybe it wasn't going to be today either. She called me and wisely suggested that we have a bit of a party—eat some chocolate, watch a funny movie, have a contraction and get back to the joy. Laugh my way through the contractions? It turned out the be the perfect advice. Nick got the kids in the car to take them to his mum's place (and had instructions to stop for copious amounts of chocolate and celebratory champagne on the way home) and I hopped into a hot bath with some music on. I sang along, enjoyed the heat of the water, and eagerly anticipated meeting our new little person.

When Nick got home, I got out of the bath and we put on a romantic comedy. I stayed on the floor contracting and pelvic rocking, hoping to turn my possibly posterior baby to get some back relief, and we laughed and had chocolate and enjoyed ourselves. Towards the end of the movie, I felt a small gush that I thought must be my water breaking (I haven't experienced it breaking before pushing so I wasn't sure) and asked Nick to fill up the birthing pool. I was excited—who knows how long now if my water has broken! But nothing really changed in the pool, and I felt no more gushing, so I decided that must have just been some other Mystery Birth Liquid. We put on some funny podcasts and just hung out, contracting and laughing. The contractions were intense. We didn't have a clock around, but we did have two other kids to keep in mind, so we had to do a bit of planning and decided that at about 7:30 p.m. Nick would go pick up our two-year-old from his mum's and bring her home (which would take about forty-five minutes), and our five-year-old would sleep over. He made sure I was okay with him leaving, and when the time came he left.

It was nice to be all alone. The contractions were still widely spaced, but very intense, and I found that when I pushed just a little bit, there was some relief from the intensity. Hmm, interesting. I kept at that, just gentle pushing for the relief when I felt like it. When Nick got back (after putting our sleeping daughter in bed) I told him he should just go hang out in another room for a while and get some rest. I was enjoying the solitude. He came and went occasionally, giving me warm top-ups in the pool, checking on whether I needed him. I continued to do my thing, listening to funny podcasts between contractions and during contractions losing myself. At one point he came and I asked him to come sit down next to the pool, and there he stayed.

I suddenly felt overwhelmed with emotion and started to cry. He asked me what was wrong, and I said that this was really hard, and I didn't want to do it anymore. He responded as he was trained to respond, "This is transition! It's almost over!" But what if it's *not* transition? Maybe I still had days ahead of me! Maybe it was going to last forever! I mentally panicked for a few seconds. I was tired. I could use a nap. Maybe I could just have a break to take a nap...? But those thoughts didn't last long. I knew I was going to have my baby in my arms soon, and that it was time to get to work.

Since I had had a cervical lip with my daughter, and since I wasn't feeling any descent and had been pushing a little bit, *and* since I was feeling a new pulling sensation with the contractions, I decided to check my cervix. I wasn't really sure what I was feeling for, but it was pretty clear once I was in there. I could feel a paper thin membrane completely across the bulging bag of waters, so I tried to push it to the side and it easily moved across. I could feel the squishy bag of waters behind it. I held the membrane to the side and pushed. The pulling sensation went away and the bag of waters started to slowly descend. I was onto something, and I kept at it until the waters had moved far enough down that the cervix wasn't an issue anymore.

Now I turned over so I was on my knees with my chest resting on Nick's lap. By now I *had* to push with each contraction whether I wanted to or not. I could feel the baby moving down, and I could see that he wasn't just going to slide out as I had assumed would happen this third time around. It was going to take some work. I continued to move him down and down and down. My waters broke with a forceful gush (eliciting a surprised "Whoa!" from both of us, and a "What was that?" from Nick who thought there must be a baby in the pool after that explosion), and from then I could feel my baby's head! I was actually touching his head!

I have no idea how long I pushed. I thought at the time, "Wow! This is almost over! This is Hard Work, but I'm doing it and he's almost here." I felt total clarity and peace.

Before long I could feel the ring of fire, and I consciously slowed things down a bit so that I wouldn't tear. His head slowly emerged with my hand still on it, guiding it. I could feel an ear on the side of his half-emerged head and said through a grunt "I can feel his ear!" (That little soft ear was the most real thing in the world at that moment, the most delicious little piece of flesh I had ever experienced. I wondered if my baby noticed that I was touching his ear while the rest of him was being squeezed so tightly. I still look at his ears now and remember that moment.) My husband wasn't in an angle to see what was happening and gave a surprised "Oh!" not realizing how far the baby had come. I could feel a shoulder under my perineum. I waited. Should I wait for the next contraction? Nah, I decided not to wait and pushed his body out with the next push.

I pulled him up out of the water which had rinsed him clean. He was a beautiful pink from what we could tell by the candlelight, and he didn't cry right away but was moving his arms and legs. I rubbed and patted his back a bit while he breathed a bit rattly, and he let out a mighty cry. He wasn't interested in breastfeeding right away and his eyes stayed closed. I asked Nick what time it was just "for the record"—10:16 p.m. "Get the camera!" Nick snapped a few pictures of us in the water. You can't see my face because I was looking down, totally absorbed in this perfect, healthy little baby that just seconds before had been inside my body.

After a few minutes the placenta came and we cut the cord. Nick wrapped Eli up in a blanket and I got out of the water and laid down under a blanket. I felt a bit lightheaded and vaguely wondered how much blood I had lost as the pool sort of resembled a crime scene. The placenta was intact so I wasn't concerned. Eli cried and cried, amazingly not waking his sleeping sister (who now looked *huge!* in comparison), maybe clearing out his lungs, maybe decompressing after this major event. I had a shower and marveled at my awesomeness.

Clean up was as easy as throwing the towels in the washing machine and emptying the pool (I had apologized to Nick in advance for how gross that was likely to be). We climbed into bed with our new person and introduced him to his amazed siblings the next morning.

And that's our story.

Matrilineal Love
Amber Magnolia

My water broke at 8:30 p.m. on Sunday, August 13th. As we ran around filling up the birthing tub and brewing anti-hemorrhage herbal teas and charging the camera, we also made sure to remember to turn our cell phones off. We set up a makeshift altar next to the tub, the centerpiece of which was the Tarot card "Trust," depicting a person free-falling or flying through empty sky, which I had pulled from the Zen Osho deck three times during the previous week. I labored through the night, switching between the birthing tub (which we had rented from the midwife), the shower, and sitting on the toilet. Every time that I had sat on the toilet during my last month of pregnancy I thought to myself that it was the ideal birth-giving position for me. Still, I wanted a water birth and spent most of my labor in the tub.

It was in this tub, during the later part of the morning of the fourteenth, that I started to periodically slip away from the assured, focused state of mind I had been in all night and began retreating into strange, dreamlike states of consciousness between contractions. I was exhausted. The baby's head was centimeters away from coming out, we could feel and see her, and I would give my all with every push, sure that with this one she would be coming out. But for what seemed like an eternity, she didn't. Still, we knew without having to verbally communicate it, that everything was all right, that our full thoughts and spirits were still in it, and that a beautiful baby would be born that day.

At about one o'clock in the afternoon we heard a tap on our front window. We were surprised and angry. Not now! Didn't they see the sign on the door? We ignored the knock. Then a few minutes later we heard rustling sounds in the back room, and shortly after that my mom and grandma entered the front room where we sat, kissing, in the birthing tub. I will never forget the moment they walked in. They seemed angelic, the afternoon sunlight dancing off the fabric of their clothes. They looked into my eyes so deeply and lovingly, and my spirit lifted and expanded. Graham and I were both renewed by their presence and the shift in energy that it brought. My grandma was crying because she had heard the sounds I was making and, as she put it, "I can't stand to see you in pain." I explained to her that it really wasn't pain so much as just a very, very intense sensation that I needed to vocalize in order to move through it.

After we caught them up on what had been happening we decided that I should get out of the tub. With the help of all three of them I made it to the bathroom, where I found relief on the toilet. The relief was short lived however because within minutes I realized that this baby was coming now! The already intense sensations became even more so, and I could feel her head crowning. Graham, who was kneeling in front of me, said, "Stand up!" and I did, bending over him and supporting myself by putting my hands on the wall there. It seemed that I was far away, projected into space; out of my body, but at the same time in it like never before.

She made sweet little sounds as her newly emerged head hung from my body, almost like a kitten mewing. Then, according to my husband, her right shoulder and then her whole right arm came out, and then the rest of her body quickly slipped into his hands. I sat back down, in awe, in shock, hand on my newly shrunken belly. "It's a girl!" said my mom, confirming the intuition that Graham and I had had all along (we always referred to the baby as "she").

We did it. It was done. Those months of anticipation, of researching and learning and discussing, of asking ourselves "are we doing the right thing?" had all culminated in this divine moment, in this unbelievably vibrant, perfect being.

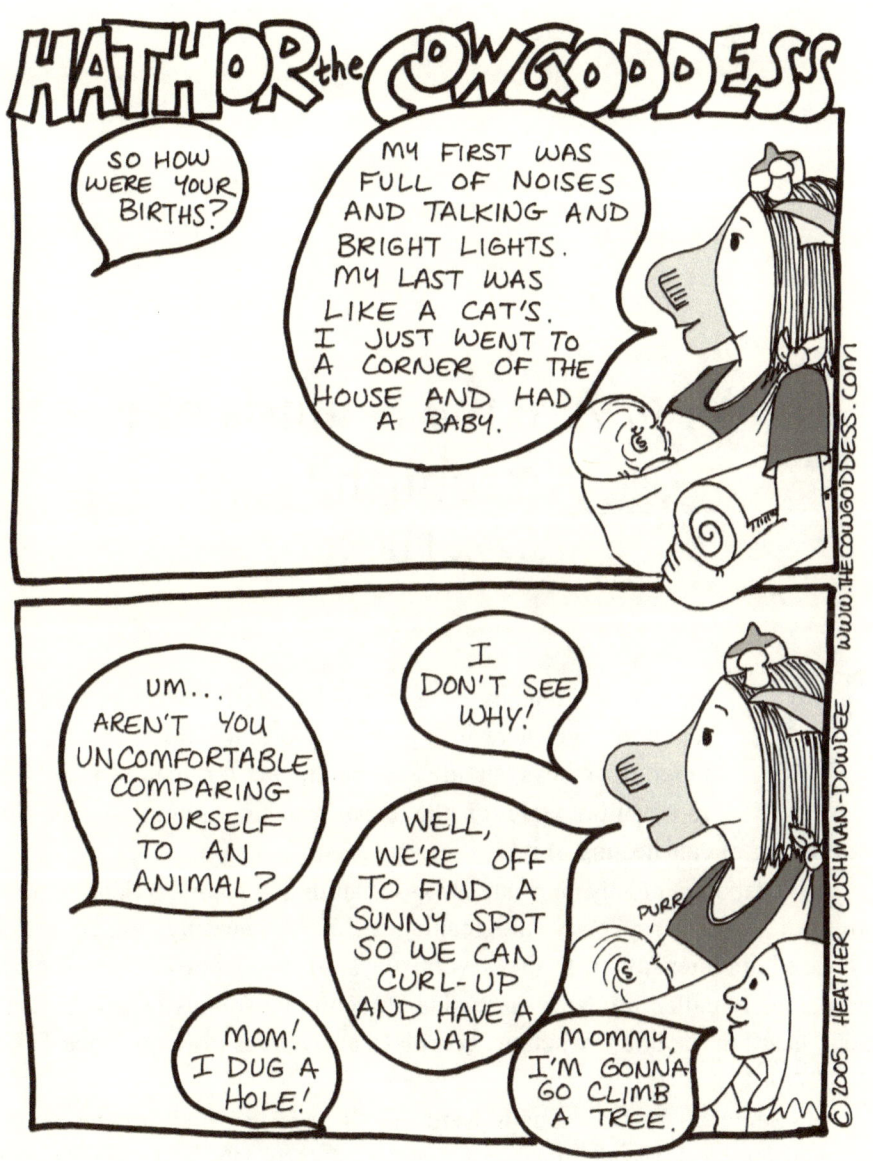

What Are the Sounds of a Freebirth?

Janet Fraser

W hat are the sounds of a home birth? In July I birthed my daughter right here in my study. Normally this room has the tapping of keys on my computer, the fortunately silent but reproachful stare of the clean washing piling up and the murmuring of cats nesting in it.

I labored mostly upright, always standing for contractions as they powered through my body and making a lot of releasing noises, which increased in intensity over the several days of my labor. In this room I inarticulately called my baby earth-side. Touchingly, sounds I made are still being heard in the house when my son plays and relives his experience of his sister's birth.

Some of the best sounds were the silences in which my supporters watched me work through each contraction. In early labour we ate lunch in the kitchen, large bowls of pasta balanced on our knees next to the wonderful island bench, friend of the home-birthing woman. When a contraction arrived I'd hand my bowl over or put it on the bench and lightly sing through it while moving my hips in the universal dance of birth. Sometimes people stopped talking, sometimes they murmured a little. I'd finish the contraction and keep eating.

In strong labor I shouted *"whoooooaaaaa,"* and stepped from foot to foot, trying to stay anchored to the world. The sounds I most needed then were loving voices around me, my son floating through now and then, his DVDs going in the background.

Even better was the sweet sound of meeting my newborn baby for the first time, hearing her birth story as she slowly blinked awake. I heard birds chatting in the dawn as my bleary-eyed support people leaned on chairs and couches and tried to stay present. I heard one of my cats who followed me from room to room, just being with me. I relished the soft splat of placenta dropping into a salad bowl before I climbed out of the pool and the creaking of springs on the futon that showed I was at last lying down to rest.

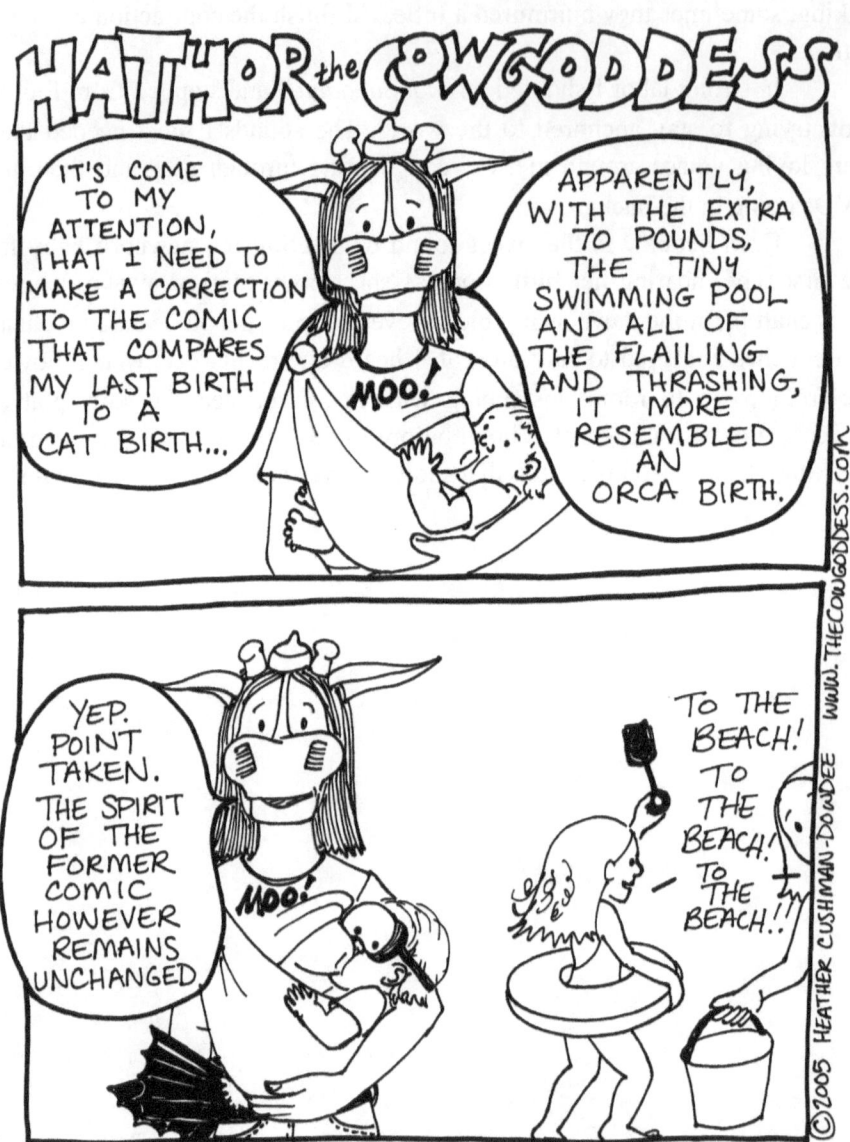

3 True Stud Rock Stars: Me, Jason and Adam

Jamie Marr Castillo

Basically to make it short, I didn't even really *know* I was in labor until 1 p.m. when I finally lost my mucous plug and things started getting more serious. I had been having contractions since 6 a.m. but they were always five minutes or more apart and not very painful at all. I did housework all day. I did several loads of laundry, put dinner in the crock-pot, scrubbed my bathroom tub and floor, vacuumed, all that stuff. But I still wasn't positive it was real labor because I hadn't lost the mucous plug and the contractions didn't seem to be getting closer together. Anyway, I did call my husband to come home from work at noon because although I wasn't sure I was in real labor, I did know that we would probably have a baby in the next day or so and I wanted him home to help take care of our daughter. At 1 p.m. when I did lose my mucous plug I thought I had hours of labor ahead of me. We called the midwife to give her a heads up. But my labor kept getting harder and harder really fast. I started getting incredibly irritated and snapped at my husband to *get out* of the bedroom. Thinking from this side of things, I should have known I was in hard active labor and entering transition, but when it's *you* and you're in the middle of it all, it is really hard to believe that things could be progressing so fast. The contractions started getting more and more intense, and I was having to breathe deeply and concentrate to get through them. I kept pacing around my bedroom like a distracted animal. It was getting harder and harder to get comfortable. At one point I tried to lie down, but I swear it hurt more. It was better to just walk walk walk the same path around my bedroom and then stop and do this toe-to-toe heel-grind dance through contractions.

Anyway, after I bit my husband's head off to *get out* of the bedroom I just started crying and sobbing. I was emotional, in pain. I decided to get into the shower to feel better. The contractions were getting so hard. I started crying out during the contractions. A primal high-pitched howl that reverberated against the shower walls. And suddenly there it was. That moment when you feel during a contraction to just relax and bulge your kegel out. Part of you wants to hold it in because you don't *want* the pain to get worse. But it's like you know, you have to do this. You must go forward. So I bulge my kegel out and there it is...the grunting. And it hurts so bad. I'm in transition and I'm grunting at the same time and I suddenly know I'm going to be having this baby soon.

I yell to Jason from the shower to *"Call Lori*!" He calls her to come. I get out of the shower and dry off and walk back into the bedroom. I'm still crying and I head over to brace myself against our dresser when another contraction comes. And it really hurts. I scream out because I just have to. I have to let it out somehow. I moan out "Jason I'm pushing...the baby is coming!" And he hears me grunt through a contraction and then he knows. This is real. This baby is coming. I tell him he needs to catch the baby. So he throws down towels and chux pads onto the floor and puts a pillow in between my feet. He asks if I can kneel down or move to the bed and I tell him, "No I can't." And it comes again. That contraction that makes you understand why women get epidurals. And then I start talking to God asking in whisper, "What is happening to me?"

My Jason said to me so calmly, "You're fine. You're fine. You're having a baby, Sweetheart. You've done this before." And then a contraction comes again, and this time when I push through it, the pushing feels good. I know the baby is moving down. I feel my skin start to stretch. I don't want to tear, so I endure the stretching. I push some more and I can feel this baby's head pushing through the center of my thighs. That *big* stretch between my legs, a pop of water...and the head is out. I can hear my husband crying with excitement telling me the head is out. I ask him to feel around the neck for a cord and he says nothing is there.

During that time when the head was out, Jason says he saw the baby's eyes were closed but the mouth would open. He thought I should hurry up and push "Eh...honey? Can you push him out?" but I knew it was okay, and I knew to wait for the contraction. When the next contraction came, I pushed the rest of his body out into Jason's hands. It was a little more than twenty minutes since I had told him to call the midwife, less than two hours after I lost the mucous plug.

We learned in that moment that we'd had a son. Something we'd waited to know. My legs were shaking. I was still standing up with the baby born behind me. I was so glad this big part was over. Adam cried the moment he came out. I could hear that he was healthy. Jason was crying. I was too tired to cry.

The baby stayed behind me for a bit as I gathered myself. We had to shuffle over to the bed and do this uncomfortable twister move to get the baby to the front of me so I could see him. *That's* when I cried, when I could see him. I was kind of worried about the placenta so I tried putting the baby to breast, but I soon started to feel another contraction and I was relieved when the placenta plopped out. I knew it was over, and we were okay.

All in all, this birth was more painful than the first, but my recovery has been unexpectedly easy. I barely tore and there was almost no blood. I had amazing energy right after birth. As for my husband and I, we just have this deeper love. I can't *wait* for my postpartum recovery to be over so I can reward him properly, ha ha!

HATHOR the COWGODDESS

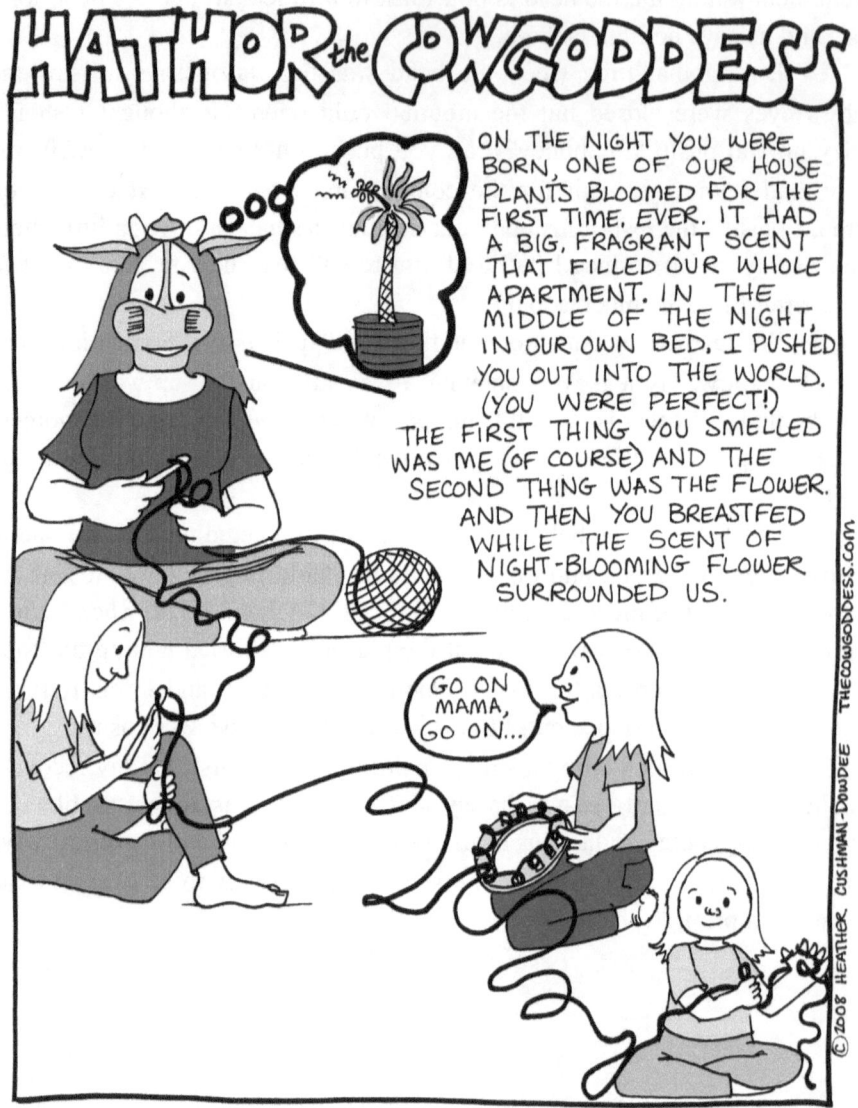

Grab the Bucket! The Baby is Coming!
Christy Lindsey

My third birth is my favorite. Since the other two were overdue, I figured this one would be, too. That is why I had decided to replace our rotten bathroom floor the week before he was due. I had spent a couple of days ripping out the old floor. My nesting instinct always seems to manifest itself in major home repairs. I went to the lumber store to get new wood for the floor. While there, I had a back pain. I hoped it wasn't labor, but I wondered. Once I got back home, I told my husband I didn't think I was in labor, but I kept having these back pains.

I remembered some acupressure points for labor that I had found on the Internet and decided to use them just in case. I could tell the difference right away. I still didn't know if I was really in labor or not but those points sure were helping.

I was in denial as it was a terrible time for the baby to decide to arrive. We had no toilet, the house was a wreck, the kids were sick, I was out of grocery staples and so on. The nest was not ready! I stayed busy doing things around the house. I cooked breakfast, cleaned a little, and worked on the bathroom floor with my husband, even getting under the house to look at boards. I just kept holding the acupressure points every time I had a back pain.

I decided if it were labor, I better blow up the pool I planned to use. I managed to get that done and had my husband hook up the hose. He had just started to fill it when I had to go outside and throw up. I came back in and had to poop, so I grabbed our temporary toilet, which was a five gallon bucket with our toilet seat on top. I sat down and my water broke. I felt the baby moving down. I told my husband to bring me the coconut oil which I then rubbed on myself to help avoid tears. I didn't push, but the baby came on down. I had three contractions. On the third one, our new son was born! My husband, covered in pressure treated sawdust caught him. He got a bulb syringe and sucked out his nose and mouth.

I sat on the bucket until after the placenta was born, and then my husband cut the cord. We were shocked the baby came so fast. Labor was less than five hours, but I didn't realize I was in labor until maybe an hour before birth. Our older son had gone outside, but the little one watched it all. He got scared by the blood, but we told him I was fine and he got in the pool to play. Our other boy came in and got in the pool. I sat on the bucket for about forty-five minutes and then got in the pool, after having the boys get out, to clean me and the baby. At least I got to use it for something! Birth is such an amazing experience. I'm so thankful to have had such an incredible birth.

Instinct and Intuition
Rebekah W.

I awoke on October 23rd around 9 a.m. with what I later figured out were labor pains. I thought I was possibly sick from something I had eaten the previous afternoon, but had a feeling that wasn't the case.

As the day progressed, the labor pains grew stronger. I soaked in the bathtub for some relief. I felt so happy and giddy that the baby was on its way. When the contractions became too strong for me to sit through, I rocked back and forth on my knees or I would lean on a chest at the foot of our bed and rock my hips back and forth.

I ate some cookies, but doing so caused me to feel like throwing up. I went upstairs and labored through increasingly stronger contractions. I leaned on the chest of drawers and rocked my hips. It felt so much better and more tolerable when I did that. The contractions felt like menstrual cramps and I considered if all of it was possibly just prodromal labor.

Each contraction was painful and immobilizing. Since using the phone was about the only thing I could do at the moment, I decided to call a friend. I described to her how I was feeling and she said that it was most likely labor, but she couldn't be sure because her contractions hadn't been the same way. Her support was encouraging and within a half-hour of the phone call my bag of waters broke.

The water breaking brought a bit of relief from the pain. From there I labored in the bathtub, mostly on hands and knees, but at times I would stand. I was concerned about exhaustion. I had slept only 4 hours the previous night. A few times I felt discouraged and worried that I wouldn't make it through without going to the hospital. I overcame those doubts by speaking encouraging things aloud and asking Chris to encourage me as well. This strengthened me and greatly improved my outlook. As labor neared the end, I took deep, long breaths to avoid hyperventilation.

Eventually I began to get urges to push, which helped give some relief from the intensity of the contractions. But the relief was short-lived and I became weary of the urges as they seemed unpredictable and uncontrollable. After a few minutes I began to feel a burning sensation and realized it as the "ring of fire" that I had seen mentioned many times.

At this point my position in the tub was hurting my knees badly. I wanted to get out and onto the bathroom floor. Chris positioned rags so there would be padding for my knees. Once I was out of the tub and on my knees I leaned far back. Laboring in this position felt great and the pushing urges were easier to deal with.

At some point I stood up and leaned on Chris' shoulders for support as he was sitting on the floor. I asked Chris a few times to check if he could see the baby's head. He said he thought he could see something. I remember touching near the opening and feeling the baby's head for the first time. It was so amazing and mysterious. We never checked station or worried about anything like that. We just went with the flow. I stood, leaning on Chris, and continued pushing. Chris got a towel ready, held it underneath me and waited while I pushed.

Without warning our baby shot out and onto the towel. It was such a relief to have him out! Chris immediately picked up our baby and turned him onto his stomach, head tilted down to clear his airways. Mucus came out of the baby's mouth and he began to cry. The sound of a baby crying in our house was so foreign to us. It felt very strange.

I don't remember what I did at that moment, other than stand there and enjoy the relief of labor being over. Chris told me it was a boy. Hearing that was very refreshing and wonderful to me. It made me happy. We were right about what we felt the whole time. Chris went into the bedroom and checked the time (our clocks were purposely kept out of sight during the last hours of labor). We estimated 12:05 a.m. as the time of birth.

At this point our baby was still crying. I sat on the toilet and latched him on to breastfeed for the first time. It was so amazing to me. I thought breastfeeding might feel uncomfortable, but it wasn't in the slightest. It was wonderful.

The baby was still fussing even while nursing and that's when we finally realized that we hadn't yet dimmed the lights—something we had planned to do as we knew how important this was for the baby during the first hours out of the womb. We quickly replaced the bright lights with the soft, soothing glow of candlelight. Within a few minutes the baby was calmly and quietly nursing. I sat there feeding him and waiting for the placenta to detach. Eventually we decided to move into the bedroom. When I stood up I found that the placenta had dropped; we placed it in a bowl with the cord still attached. We then moved the baby, the placenta bowl and ourselves into our bed while I continued to feed the baby. I don't remember how long he nursed, but at some point he finished and was resting peacefully. While our baby slept I looked at him closely for the first time. I was in awe of how beautiful and perfect he was. Chris and I laid there and admired our baby for quite a while. Then we too joined him in rest..

Simple, Everyday Miracles: Rowan's Birth
Jennifer S. Bax

I had been in the shower for maybe ten minutes when I got out to tell him that I needed the pool *now*. And I promptly went and got into it. The pool was set up in my living room, and was about a quarter filled. John had started working on it as soon as I came home and informed him that my waters had released. We never did get a hose or an attachment for the faucet, so he was filling it one bucket at a time. Luckily, we had a wonderful hot water heater, it never failed me. And John boiled pot after pot of water (how stereotypical can you get?) to "hot up" my pool even more.

When the pool was about two-thirds full of blissfully hot water, John set up camp in the living room. He dragged in the mattress from our son's (unused) toddler bed, covered it with sheets and a comforter, and tried to go back to sleep, while I labored in the pool. It was about midnight. I'd made John turn the clock away from me, because I didn't want to watch it all night. I knew I had a long slog ahead, and I didn't want to get discouraged. I'd seen that the contractions were coming roughly every 2 minutes, and I didn't want to know any more.

The contractions... I'm not sure what to say about them. In the shower, I handled them best by letting the water spray on my back, down low (where I kept my fists jammed most of the night, so much so that my shoulders were killing me the next day) while I rocked my hips back and forth. I was chanting the Goddess Chant through each surge—Isis Astarte Diane Hecate Demeter Kali Inanna—Isis Athena Rhiannon Cerridwen Brid Anath Arianrhod.

Soon it changed to "Open" over and over, longer and more drawn out with each surge: "Ooooooooopennnn. Ooooooooooooooppppppennnnnnn." Four or five of those got me through a contraction.

In the pool, early on, I spent time on my knees, still rocking my pelvis. When a contraction came, I had to submerge—get under it, literally. I went to my hands and knees, then into a push-up position. I hung onto the side of the pool, chanting "open" again and again—my old trick of counting through each contraction, which I used throughout my labor with Gareth during an idiotic seventeen-hour induction, failed me this time. Nor was I able to escape the sensations and go elsewhere, the way I had last time. This was much faster, much more intense.

I found I was better able to handle the contractions on my feet, so I stood up much of the time, knee-deep in warm water, fists thrust into the hollow of my back, toning. "Open" was now just "Ohhhhhh...ohhhhhhh" low and loud. I couldn't control it, though I didn't want to wake John up. I stood there in the semi-darkness, the living room lights were out, but the bathroom light shone through; singing my birth song and trying to work with, rather than against, the expansions of my uterus.

And so I labored. As before, I had no concept of time. John tells me it was about 1 a.m. when my vocalizing changed and he woke up fully (he'd only been dozing anyway). About 1:30 he remarked casually, "They're less than a minute apart now. You *are* progressing. They're lasting about twenty seconds."

Twenty seconds? I was crushed. I kept thinking, "Longer, stronger, closer together." If these were only twenty seconds!

"I don't want to know that," I groaned. "Don't tell me that."
A small piece of my mind wondered where I was, dilation-wise. I didn't want to psych myself into thinking it would be done soon, even though it felt *very* fast and intense to me. I was trying to prepare myself, physically and mentally, for another whole day of this—longer, if necessary! There were clues, and I couldn't help but notice them: the way I was toning through contractions, the lowing, birth-song quality to them. Shorter, more intense contractions could mean I was in or near transition. I was starting to feel

89

nauseated at the end of each surge. I never did throw up, but I told John repeatedly that I felt I might. I started dozing or "zoning out" between contractions, drifting into a strange, incoherent "laborland." I could only endure contractions by standing and rocking my hips, then getting underwater and floating once I'd passed the peak.

I realized I was feeling very foggy. Random thoughts crossed my mind: bizarre, dreamlike notions that seemed to make sense at the time, even though a part of me knew they didn't.

Then, abruptly, the fog lifted. Suddenly I was thinking clearly again, the world came back into focus. And to my astonishment and chagrin, I realized that I was pushing at the end of each contraction!

This can't be right, I thought wildly. Something's wrong, it's too soon.

But it didn't feel wrong; it felt right. Not good, but *right*. So I pushed.

I remember thinking, I want this over! I want it over and done. How much can a person be expected to take? This is silly! I did not have to do this, I could've signed up for a repeat c-section!

I don't think I said any of this aloud, but I know I did whine, "I can't do this!" once or twice. John came and looked me straight in the eyes, saying, "Yes, you can, you are, you're doing great." I reminded myself that I'd known what I was getting into, I'd made my choices and I had to accept them, and whinging about it wasn't going to help anything. I may as well be there, since I had to be. It was like that old kids' game, *Going on a Bear Hunt*: "Can't go over it. Can't go under it. Have to go *through* it."

The urge to push was subtle. It wasn't "I gotta *push*," the way it was when I was laboring with Gareth. It was like something had taken over my body and was pushing whether I liked it or not! I began to roar with each push, getting louder and stronger.

"You're progressing," John said with satisfaction.

"I think I'm pushing," I told him.

"Don't wear yourself out. Take it easy."

Easy to say, but the effort was impossible to resist. I was worried, it still seemed too early (as far as I can make out, it was only about 2 a.m.) to be pushing. I hadn't been laboring long enough. I was afraid that I was only five centimeters with a badly mal-positioned baby, that I was making it worse with every surge, swelling my cervix and sealing my doom. I didn't know what to do, and I said so. Then, in a fit of desperation and doubt, I asked John to check me, the first vaginal exam I'd had since I was nine weeks along and worried about a possible miscarriage.

He went and scrubbed up. Offered to use bleach(!!!), but I convinced him that soap and water was sufficient, as long as he scrubbed for at least twenty seconds. (I think he did two solid minutes.) He came back, and we waited through another contraction. Then I tried to lay back and let him fumble around for a moment or two, as long as I could endure. He reported, "No, nothing."

I wanted to cry. In fact, I think I did cry, a little it. How much more could I bear? What should I do?

Another surge, like a terrier shaking a rat. Lots of show, some gushing fluid, intense pressure in my rectum. Something was moving through me, there was no escaping it. "It feels like it's right there," I kept saying. "It" was hard to describe, but it felt foreign, not me. It seemed to move opposite to me. If I swung my hips left, it rotated right, or else I rotated around it while it stayed still. It didn't hurt, but it was very, very uncomfortable. There was no getting away from it. It was...inexorable.

I pushed and roared and pushed, giving up my brain's worries to let my body, my primitive self, take over. "I surrender," I told the Universe. "Whatever happens..."

It went on, and on, and on. I had no clue what time it was, or how long I'd been there. I pushed standing up in my pool until my knees shook and threatened to buckle, then I went back to kneeling. I tried to push while lying on my side, first right, then left, but while floating on my side and back between contractions felt good, pushing in those position did *not!*
Standing was best. Kneeling was tolerable, but only just. Sitting, lying, even floating in the push-up pose I'd used earlier, these were all completely untenable. Surge, push, howl like a wolf. Repeat.

Push. Roar! Breathe. Again. And again. Have I ever worked so hard in my life?

Push. Push with all my might. I was worried that I was doing the "purple pushing" encouraged in hospitals. Shouldn't I be trying to breathe the baby out instead?

Screw it! I thought grimly. I don't care if I tear six ways from Sunday. I want this kid out!

Push. Roar! Breathe.

Over and over, more than body and soul can bear. I can't do it. I can't. Not anymore. I can't.

"Yes, you can," John insisted. "You've come this far. You're not giving up now. You've told me a hundred thousand times you can do it, and I believe you. You *can*."

I reached down, trying to see if I could feel...something, anything. "If it helps," John was saying, "your belly [meaning the bump that was Rowan] is lower." With my last push, I had felt a stinging sensation, and the phrase "ring of fire" had danced through my mind, but I had quickly dismissed it. Still, maybe my perineum was at least bulging a bit.

And there "it" was, just under my fingers, barely inside me: a squishy soft mound, damp and warm. I froze. O my dear good Goddess!

"There's a head there," I said, shocked.

Another push—the head slipped back, but only a little, and there was a definite burn now. I didn't care—it wasn't bad, and anyway, there was a head there! Set me on fire, I don't mind. I'm *birthing*!!

The surge ended. "Want to feel?" I asked John, and he reached into the water—I must have been kneeling at this point. I can't describe the expression on his face. "Yeah," he whispered. "Yeah..."

PUSH! I bore down hard, pressing my fingers hard into the skin around my vagina, trying to stretch the tissues. That one stung—but in the next moment, I had a small(!) firm head in my hand! John was holding it too. Rowan was out to his ears, maybe, and I was yelling. It *hurt*, the only part of the whole labor I could truthfully call, well, excruciating.

"What now?" John wanted to know. He was stunned.

"Wait," I gasped, "for the next contraction..."

"Come on..."

It felt like forever. I tried to push without the contraction, but the baby didn't budge. For the first time all night I was praying, pleading, *begging* for another contraction!

Finally it came, and I *pushed*.

The head came out; the shoulders and body quickly followed. (So much for my fears about shoulder dystocia!) Before my brain could register was had happened, I was holding a slippery new baby in my arms!

I sat back in the pool, which up till now had stayed remarkably clear, was now murky with fluid, blood, mucus, and fecal material. But it was mine; there was no meconium. I didn't care what I was sitting in. I had done it! *I birthed my baby*!!!!

"Hello," I crooned to my new little bug. "Oh, hello!"

He was perfect (well, I didn't know he was a "he" yet) snuggled up to my shoulder. He was dusky, but his face and chest were pink. He hadn't made a sound. I rubbed him, talked to him. He opened his eyes and looked at me, but he still didn't make a peep.

"Hi, sweetie," I said. "Oh, you're so beautiful. Look at you, oh, hello, Rowan!"

He finally whimpered a little when I gave into John's increasingly anxious requests and turned him over to check the sex. I laughed in surprise: "Oh my God, it's Rowan Riley!"

I couldn't stop thinking, I did it! I *did* it!! *I did it!!!!!*

"What time...?" I managed.

"Congratulations!!!" John shouted. "You did it! 4:33 a.m.!"

4:33 a.m.? That's *all*?! I was in complete shock—my water broke at 5 p.m., I'd only really labored since 11 p.m. Five and half hours, and most of it pushing...? Early in the evening I had joked, "Wouldn't it be great if the kids could wake up and find their new sibling? And I could call my mom and tell her to stop by on her way to work?" I never thought it would happen...

Birth happens. I know it does. It happened right there in a blowup pool in my living room. Birth happens. It wasn't perfect, I still had a retained placenta to deal with. But in the end, it was all so beautifully simple. Rowan was born, and so was I.

Ari's Birth
Seraf

One Wednesday afternoon in August, as predicted by my two-year-old, subtle cramps began coming at seven minute intervals. My partner wanted to call off work, but I sent her anyway, "What could happen in three hours?"

We dawdled and played and finally made our way out the door for the nap-time stroll. The walk was a short one, only around one block. I sang Osha a song about the baby we would be meeting that night. I had a couple of contractions on the first side of the square route and several more on the final side. I joked with a neighbor that I was moving slower or the contractions were coming faster, but I couldn't be sure which it was.

Once home, I went to take a bath. I climbed into the water and the contractions immediately stopped. I laughed to myself that I hadn't wanted to relax that much. The phone rang; I hopped out. Sales call. I politely declined and resumed my bath. My contractions began again with an intensity they had previously lacked. Lamenting my lack of birth classes this pregnancy, I called the midwives' office to ask for advice about comfort measures. They were gone, so I just got back in the bath.

I got the sensation that my body was pushing and got out to check my dilation. I'd never been able to reach my cervix in the past, and now it felt so close. It felt like there was no opening, but eventually I realized it extended to the far reaches of my fingertips. My fingers were spread as far apart as they could go without difficulty. Oh. I jumped up to find a tape measure with centimeters. Seven. Not enough to push, but my body will do as she pleases. The phone rang again, this time a cousin. I told him I was in labor and to please not visit. He chided, "Why are you answering the phone if you're in labor?" It finally occurred to me to bring the cordless phone. It rang again, my mom, and again, my partner, Jen. She was coming home, she'd gotten lost twice on the way to work and felt like being home with me. "Would you pick me up some juice?" I'd asked. She would not, but she would delegate a friend to bring me some.

I moved into the bedroom, where the air conditioner was running. Jen arrived to find me laying with my knees on the floor and my head on the bed. She asked what to do, I pointed out the birth kit and asked for a popsicle. She brought me a popsicle, called the midwives, readied the birth kit and brought in the birthing stool Osha and I had made. It was a five-gallon bucket with the front quarter cut out. There was about four inches of bucket at the bottom, and a large U-shaped opening above. On top, the throne was a toilet seat with the front removed. Osha and I had painted it with bright patches. The creation was an amusing form of nesting.

Jen's face was white, and I laughed at her nervousness. She pointed out that a lot had changed in the hour and a half she was gone. I sat on the birth stool because my bowels felt like moving and I didn't feel like running into the bathroom. Nothing new happened and I checked myself again. There was no head, but the bag of waters just inside. "This feels really cool!"

Jen looked at me funny and said, "I'm going to wash my hands." She was still dressed in her work clothes. When she returned, ghostly pale, "I can see the head."

I laughed and reached to find the crown myself. Jen squatted in front of me with the next contraction. I tried not to push. With a pop Ari exploded from me. She made impact like a football into Jen's arms before being thrust into my own. Her wails assured us she could breathe. I untangled her cord from her leg and neck before I could find her face. Jen dried her off. Then, as if remembering her nervousness, jumped back and almost shouted, "What do I do?"

"How about a blanket?" Still smiling, I glanced at the clock and we marveled at how quickly it had happened. The first contraction had been less

95

than 4 hours earlier. Osha had been asleep less than an hour. Jen had only been home half an hour before Ari arrived.

I've been told she was born in the caul, and that means she'll be lucky. I'm not sure about that, though I know she'll be among the fortunate who know birth is safe and natural.

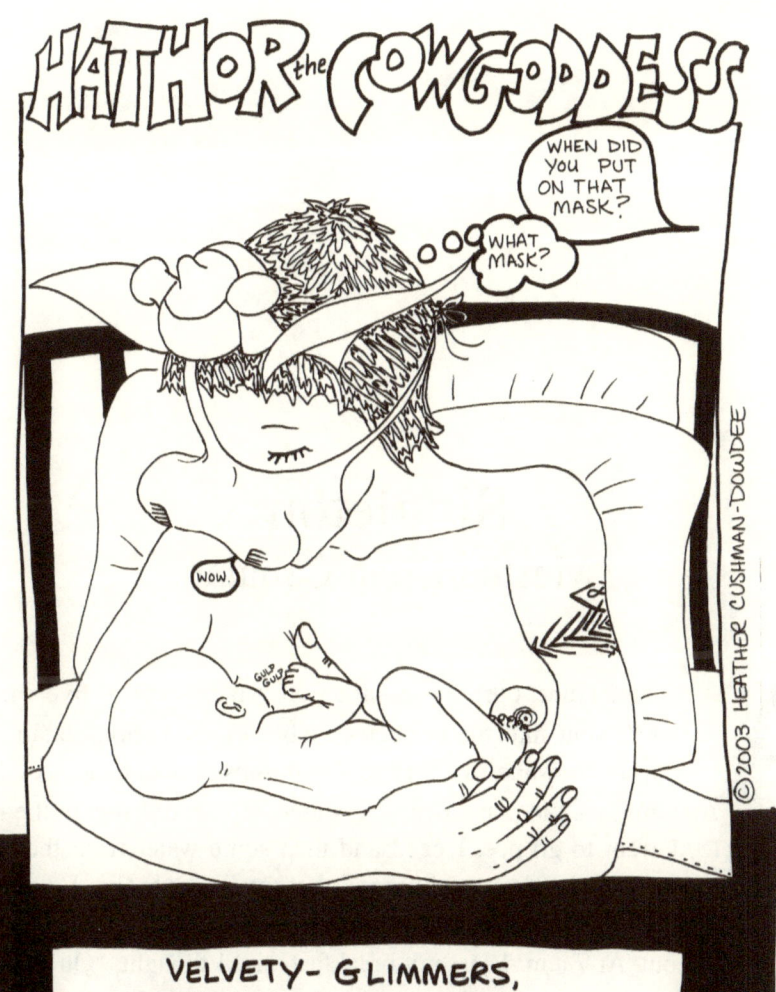

VELVETY- GLIMMERS,
CAREENING CARESSES.
YOU. INDELIBLY ETCHED
WHERE NOTHING EXISTED BEFORE.

Singleton
Martha Ellen Cahalan

At 1 a.m. (June 6th) my contractions started being five minutes apart. I went into the kitchen to labor in my rocking chair. I did not want to wake my husband and sons. I spent the wee hours rocking, walking, and drinking water. Whatever I was in the mood for. At 5:15, I went to go pee. I peed and then some water from the wrong hole gushed out. I shouted to my husband that my water broke. I went back to the rocking chair. I still had a lot of water, because with each contraction more gushed out. At 7 a.m. I lost my breakfast, and I thought, "Oh good, it's almost over." At 9 a.m. my husband woke the kids. I told him not to. At 10 a.m., my husband, Albert, was chasing the kids around the house. I was feeling pushy. I was also starting to worry if the baby was stuck. Albert reassured me that he is not stuck.

At 11 a.m., Albert took the kids outside. After a while, Albert came back and noticed that he could see the baby's head. I pushed and out came his head. Albert said that he looks a little blue. I checked for a cord around his neck. I loosened the cord and pushed out his shoulders. Then the rest of him fell out. Within a few moments he started to cry. About a half hour later I squatted to deliver the afterbirth.

Still today, my husband, Albert, says this was our best birth yet.

Twins!
Martha Ellen Cahalan

A round 2:30 a.m. my husband got into bed. He was on the computer. I was a good girl, I went to bed at 10 p.m. To give him space, I move over. *Pop!* "I think my water broke!" Never mind, perhaps it is my imagination. I start to lie back down. Wetness. My water did break! We lay down a shower curtain on the carpet of our bedroom.

I am having contractions. Labor can take hours. I've only had four hours of sleep. My husband had none. We decide to go back to bed. He will try to sleep on the floor, while I labor in bed. The contractions get stronger. So strong that I hope they will not get any more stronger. I am still expecting hours of labor left. I have to go to the bathroom. I waddle to the toilet. Once I am in front of the toilet, I get the sudden urge to vomit. (If I had had the urge sooner I would run, not walk, to the bathroom.) Of course, I vomit into the toilet. I sit on the toilet. I pee and poop. I get the sudden desire for needing my husband to be near me.

I call for my husband. He does not come. I crawl back to the bedroom and shout for him to wake up. He wakes up with a start. I have an involuntary pushing urge. Then Fiona's head crowns. My husband takes a few pictures and catches her. 5:13 a.m.

I pick up my new daughter. I try to nurse her. The contractions hurt too much to be just a placenta in me. Something is not right. I complain to my husband. He cuts the cord to Fiona. I move back into the bathroom. I am in a kneeling squat, using the edge of the bathtub for support. I give strong voluntary pushes. The "placenta" feels hard and bony.

My husband sees a bulge coming out. He prepares to deliver the "placenta." He sees an awfully big and featureless bag full of icky juice. He spies an ear. This is not a placenta. It is another baby still in her caul. I give a huge push. The bag breaks. My husband catches Melanie.

Melanie is not breathing. I tell my husband to start rescue breathing. (Reminding him to use only the air in his cheeks.) My husband gives only two breaths and gives up. I take Melanie from him and tell him to get a book for me. I continue rescue breaths. My husband fails to notice that I put post-it notes to mark places in the book that might be needed in a hurry. He looks up "Infant Resuscitation" in the index. I notice a pulse in her cord. (Duh, my high school CPR class did not tell me to check for a pulse there.) Melanie starts to take breaths on her own. My husband instructs me to talk to Baby B and keep her warm. I tell her to "Keep breathing!"

Melanie's breathing and color improves. Things are stable. We should have Melanie checked out by our family pediatrician. After arranging child care for our sons, we take the girls to the pediatrician. Both girls are fine.

The Unassisted Water Birth of Khéna Maël

Melissa Bellemare

The week before Khéna was born was full of false starts. He twisted and turned inside of me, but he wouldn't engage at all... During the day, evening and night of the 27th of November, the contractions were different, though. They woke me up, but they were far apart or came in spurts. I thought that it was the start. I also had a bit of mucous and I was a bit more dilated and during the night he had made his way back into the optimal LOA (Left Occiput Anterior) position and I was feeling a lot more pressure on my cervix.

So when Simon offered to stay home from work I was completely open to it. However, soon after I got up, the contractions subsided again. I felt discouraged; I felt bad that I had made Simon stay home again. I was tired of the false starts.

The contractions kept coming at about six to seven minute intervals. With the contractions came pressure. They were not painful per say but were uncomfortable. I could talk through them, but I had to lift myself a bit off the chair with each one because of the pressure on my cervix and pelvic floor. I walked around, sat down, went on the computer and wondered if it were the real thing and wondered if I should fill up the pool.

I decided that it would be a good idea and if ever it were just another false alarm then I would at least be comfortable in the warm water. I changed position often, the pressure that came with each contraction was starting to become hard to deal with. In my mind, however, I was not yet sure that it was it, but I couldn't wait to hop into the pool. By the time that there was enough water in the pool, the hot water had run out. But though it was not warm enough yet I couldn't wait, and I hopped in while Simon started to boil water to heat the pool up more.

Simon sat down at the computer to write this:

"The contractions have been getting stronger and stronger ever since the middle of the afternoon. I recognize the expression on Melissa's face when she gets them; she looks far away, deep down in the faraway depths of her own body and psyche. Right here and now; carpe diem; no way around it. It's the look that means she's really in labor now; it surely isn't a false alarm.

She's in the pool now, in the middle of the living room, and I closed the blinds and turned off the phones. Shut off against the world. I'm boiling pot after pot of water to make the water just right"

I was expecting the contractions to stop at that point but instead, they kept on coming. I took them on one at a time and tried to distract myself with the new movie that the boys were watching. Soon though, I couldn't handle the noise of the movie anymore. It was distracting, but I didn't need to be distracted anymore. I needed to go inside myself at that point.

It was about 6:40 p.m. by then; the contractions were taking up all of my attention, and I needed to change position often in the pool. Breathing though them was no longer enough and now I needed to moan and growl. I found positions that worked for a few contractions and eagerly awaited each pot of hot water that Simon brought. The water temperature was good and the water was keeping warm in the birthing pool, but the extra hot water each time just felt great for the next contraction. I floated in the water, kneeled, laid on my side and just let the contractions come.

By about 7 p.m. the contractions were one on top of the other. I felt like jumping out of my skin. My brain was separated into two voices: one that was in the moment and was panicking and wanted to jump out the window and the other that knew that everything was normal and never let the other lose control. I reached inside to see how things were and if I could feel the head, and I was discouraged for a second when I couldn't feel it. Then I felt something in a place that I didn't expect and then realized that the head was right there but just not where I thought it would be; he was closer than I thought. I felt the edge of the cervix and knew that it wouldn't be too long.

With the next contraction I tried to push a bit and it felt so good. At that moment I got a break. I was able to talk and regroup a bit. I told Simon to give Colin his bath. I let the contractions keep on coming and asked Simon to get the bed ready in case I wanted to try braving the contractions on dry land and then told Simon that I had felt the head when he passed by.

The contractions kept on coming and my moans and growls were no longer good enough and now a louder voice escaped my body at the peak of each contraction.

At 7:35, I felt the need to push a bit, and when I did my water broke… I felt relief again and for a minute or two and again I was given a break. I asked Simon to pour hot water on my back. When my body went back into action it was the end, I felt out of control, a massive cramp struck the muscles in my side, my mind shifted from the contraction to the cramp. The contraction went away, and I was able to change position to get rid of the cramp and then the next contraction hit. I was in control again, and I felt that unmistakable need to push; waves came over my body. I knew that it was the end, so I called out to Simon. Each wave brought the head closer and closer, my body pushed, and I helped it, but it knew exactly what to do without my help. I said to tell Xavier as the head emerged. The contraction then stopped, and I waited for the next while I stroked his head. The next contraction came, and he stayed put while I pushed. Simon suggested I kneel, but my body decided to go on all fours and he came out. As I turned back around Simon was pulling him out of the water and announced that he was a boy. We got the cord unwrapped from around his neck and waited for him to breathe. He was quiet, his body was a beautiful pink but his head was still purple. I patted his back and tried a few different positions and then a sense of calm came over me. I knew he was okay. He opened one eye a bit, looked at me, whimpered, and then closed it again. He was sleeping. I felt the placenta pool up around my cervix, I gave one slight push and it just flowed out into the pool water. It was 7:45, and I was holding my third son. He was nameless, but I was in love.

Simon took a few pictures while the boys met their new brother. The first words to come out of Colin's mouth were: "Baby! He's so cute." I asked Simon to bring me a bit of Shepherd's Purse tincture, as I couldn't see how much blood was in the pool, and then I asked him to bring me the bowl for the placenta.

We wrapped our beautiful new baby up in a warm towel in his father's arms and juggled both the baby and the bowl with the Placenta. I got out of the pool and we all went to the bedroom to welcome the new baby more comfortably. Simon and I then spent a few minutes recapping the events of the evening and admired our third son and finally gave him his name. Khéna was not a name that we had really contemplated but it was on one of the lists that Simon had made. While looking at each name on the lists it stood out in a way that it had not before. It fit. It is a South American name that means "little flute of the Indes" and it is pronounced "Kay-na."

About four hours after he was born, we cut his cord. It was thin, though the placenta was healthy and big. We put him in a shirt and a dry warm blanket and he slept.

Amazing, Simple, Extraordinary
Stephanie Whalen

I was still feeling crampy and contracting and having a lot of bloody show, though I still didn't know if birth was around the corner or a ways off. Everybody went to bed and I got up around 1 a.m. like I had been for the past few days because I was unable to sleep through my contractions (they got worse at night). I watched TV and went online for a bit and tried to doze. The contractions got stronger and started coming about every seven minutes or so. They were only lasting about thirty-seconds though.

I was trying to figure out what I was going to do about Pat and work. This labor and pregnancy had been so different from what I was used to that I still wasn't really sure about whether the baby was going to come or if the contractions were going to taper off and we would have to wait another day. In the end I decided that I would tell him that I wanted him to stay even though I couldn't guarantee that we would have a baby by the end of the day. I waited for 6 a.m. when his alarm was going to go off and then I was going to tell him. By the time 6 a.m. rolled around, I didn't even add anything about not being sure, I just told him that I wanted him to stay. At that point my contractions were bad enough that I was breathing hard through them.

As soon as I got up and started trying to move around and do stuff, things really really picked up. I had maybe six or seven or eight contractions that just took my breath away while I was in the shower, drying off, and getting prepared. I set everything up in front of the love-seat so that I could lean over it during contractions. I also brought out the candle that I had burned on the night of my grandmother's funeral and put it on top of the entertainment center and lit it up. I needed it there because I knew she was going to help guide the baby into the world.

I settled onto the floor and alternated for a while between having contractions on all fours on the floor and leaning over the couch. I was trying very hard to relax my stomach muscles while I was contracting because that hurt less, but it was a difficult thing to do. I grabbed a blanket at some point and draped it over myself because I was uncomfortable with my bare butt hanging out (go figure). Eventually, I was only wanting to be leaning over the couch while I was contracting. The contractions were getting very intense. I started vocalizing some when they came. As one came on, I would start breathing hard and blowing, then moan or scream, then move back to breathing hard or blowing, then trying to catch my breath again when it was over. It was probably about 7:30 at this point. Saren came out when I was still leaning over the couch. She looked at me and seemed groggy and a bit awestruck.

I was getting very tired. I started thinking that I just wanted to go to sleep and that I just wanted a little break to nap for a while and then I could do it again. I kept remembering when I was in the hospital with Saren and Harper and how with each of them I had been given Stadol, which made me sleep in between contractions. I was remembering how I had been lying on my side back then, and I couldn't stop thinking how good it would feel to just lay down. So I asked for a blanket to use as a pillow and I laid down on my left side, just as I had been in the hospital. It did feel good to lie down, but the contractions didn't slow down and I didn't get any break. I think I almost thought that just the act of lying down would make my body take a break. The contractions were still very strong. I decided to start really vocalizing through them, really yell. While doing that I was thinking about how I hadn't done so with Saren or Harper, maybe because I just felt much more inhibited in the hospital, I'm not sure. I remember feeling really free while yelling and just thinking, "Go ahead and scream. Nobody's going to stop you." I did, and Harper woke up and came out. She says she was plugging her ears, but I don't remember that. She laid down next to me in between a contraction and I rubbed her back a little and held her. She asked for some cereal and I told her that I couldn't get it for her, and she started to look very upset and like she wanted to cry.

Pat started walking with her to the kitchen to get her some cereal, but before they were there, a contraction started up and I felt my water break in a gush. Right on top of that was a huge, overwhelming, uncontrollable urge to push. Not even really an urge to push, my body just kind of started pushing. I was nervous because I was lying on my side and my legs were together and I didn't feel very much like I could move into any kind of good position for the baby to come. I had wanted to be more upright. I said, "Pat! I need you!" He came over and I could tell he didn't know what was going on (I was actually still covered by a blanket) and I could only say, "Baby!" I pulled the cover off and said, "Need up!" He helped me pull my upper body into more upright position and to lift my leg and I could feel the baby moving down and my body pushing her, pushing, pushing. It felt so good to push. She was moving out fast. It only took a couple of pushes till she was crowning and then a few more to get her completely out. Probably less than a minute from when I said, "Pat" to when she was out. Ironically, my thoughts about laying down and the hospital turned out to be a good thing because she shot out so fast. I'm afraid if I had been on hands and knees she just would have slipped through Pat's hands and fallen onto the floor.

I immediately saw that she was a girl and was a bit disappointed about it. Not that she was a girl, but that my intuition was so off. Pat said, "It's a girl," and we were both holding her slippery, warm, wet little body in our hands. She was immediately pink; I don't remember her being purple at all. She cried right away, but was a bit gurgly, so I had Pat put her on my leg on her tummy and we both rubbed her back for a few seconds. The cord was very short and we couldn't bring her up to my chest, so I sent Pat off for some scissors and the string that I had made to tie off her cord. I had intended on not cutting it, but since it was so awkward and she was breathing perfectly, we went ahead and tied it off and cut it.

I waited for the placenta and honestly thought it would come right away. However, it took two full hours. During that time, I held the baby a bit and tried to nurse her, but she wasn't very interested. She was very alert and very calm. She didn't cry anymore after having done so initially. She just looked around at everybody. Pat and the girls held her more during this time than I did because I was so very uncomfortable from the placenta not having been delivered yet. I tried just pushing every so often over a bowl, but it just wasn't coming. It just needed a little bit of time (and some very uncomfortable contractions) to detach itself. Finally, after a biggish crampy contraction, I felt like it was ready and I pushed it into the bowl. I felt a million times better.

I took a shower and cleaned the baby a little bit, put a diaper on her and finally called my mother.

All in all, it was amazing. It was the most amazing and simple and extraordinary thing I've ever done. I'm thrilled with myself, and I'm thrilled with this birth.

Arissa's Birth Story
Kelly Silliman

After my blessingway ended, around 9:30 p.m., I was standing talking to my mom when I felt a sudden wetness in my underwear. I excused myself, not knowing if it was my water breaking, and when I went to the bathroom, I realized it was my mucus plug. I also had some bloody show. I started to need dark and quiet during contractions, which were speeding up in intensity and frequency rather quickly. I would go into the spare bedroom and get on my hands and knees or child's pose on the bed and breathe through them. Then I got nauseous, so I went to the bathroom and threw up. I had a few contractions on my hand and knees on the bathroom floor. At one point, Rosalie came in, asking me what was going on. I had heard people explaining to her that the baby was coming soon, and so I just said, "I need you to put your hand on my back and be quiet." She put her hands gently on my back and just whispered "what" very softly over and over, not really expecting an answer. It was exactly what I needed.

After that I went back to the bedroom. I started humming through my contractions, and wanted people out of my house so I could make more noise and take my clothes off. My mom came in to say goodbye, but I was in the middle of a contraction, and I think I said, "Don't come in. I love you. Go away."

I started opening my mouth and really vocalizing through the contractions. They were getting stronger and stronger and much closer together. I kept alternating between hands-and-knees and side-lying positions. I couldn't stay in one position for very long, which was so different from last time. I wanted to rest in between contractions, but they were so close together, I only had time to change position or rest, not both. Finally Tom and Rosalie came in to be with me. The first thing I said was "Get these pants off of me!" I wanted to be naked (another change from my last labor). Tom and Rosie would bring me water when I asked, but there was nothing I really wanted them to do. At one point, I asked Tom to put his hands on my lower back. I was feeling the contractions in my lower abdomen, reaching around to the back of my pelvis. But when Tom climbed on the bed, the movement was unbearable so I told him to get off. A little bit later, Tom asked me to tell him when I hit transition. I yelled, "There's not going to be a transition!" Things were pretty intense at this point.

I was starting to feel pushy, but I also needed to poop. I reached down to see if I could feel a head, and there was nothing in the birth canal, so I figured I had time to get to the bathroom. I asked Tom to help me stand up. As soon as I stood I could feel my body bearing down. I started to poop, so I yelled "Get the poop! Get the poop!" Tom sort of knocked it out of the way, and then I yelled, "The head!" and squatted down. By the time I squatted the head was about a third of the way out and I could feel the "ring of fire." I also felt like I might have a small tear near the top of my canal. I started saying, "Gentle, Chickpea" over and over while stroking the head and waiting for the next contraction. Tom was next to me, and Rosalie was crouched in front of me watching the baby's head. Pushing didn't feel as good this time as it had with Rosalie, but with the next contraction, the rest of the head came out, and then almost immediately, the body. I caught the baby as it came out, and I saw fluid gush out of the nose and mouth. The baby began to cry right away, and so I offered my breast. The baby latched on pretty quick, and nursed almost constantly for the next three hours.

I looked right away to see if it was a boy or a girl, and in the very dim light of the bedroom, I thought it was a boy. But when I checked a second time, I realized we had a baby girl! I was so thrilled. I had always wanted two girls. But we had no idea what we were going to name her! We looked at the time and realized that the baby had been born about ten minutes before 11 p.m., less than an hour and a half after I lost my plug. No wonder labor had been so intense! She came out pretty clean, with no vernix on her (just like Rosalie) but with quite a bit of blood on her head.

About half an hour after the baby was born, I birthed the placenta. It came out but stayed attached by the membranes so it was hanging between my legs. I stayed squatting as long as I could, but the thing would not come out, so I got up on the bed to wait. During the next few hours I nursed, and rested as Tom and my friends cleaned up and called people and took care of Rosalie.

I wanted to wait until the placenta was entirely out before cutting the cord, but after three hours I really had to pee. I tried to squat while Tom held the placenta behind me so I wouldn't pee on it and Mary Catherine held a bucket between my legs. (Really, really good friends!) But every time I tried to do this, the baby would cry (I was holding her and she was still attached) and I couldn't concentrate. Finally we decided to just go ahead and cut the cord. I was still having trouble peeing while squatting over the bucket, and I couldn't go to the toilet because of the placenta, so I decided to just pee on the chux pad. We had several underneath me, and I had peed when I lost my plug, so I thought it would be fine. Once I started peeing, however, fluid just gushed out of me and didn't stop. Mary Catherine was there, and we started laughing, and she asked me if my water had ever broken. I said, "Well, it must have, since she wasn't born in the caul, but it never really gushed out." She said, "This must be your waters because I don't think this much pee is possible." It filled two or three chux pads and then made a huge puddle on the floor. I think that the membranes must have been holding the waters inside until then.

We decided to weigh and measure the baby, because she seemed smaller than Rosalie had been and I had been expecting this one to be bigger. We couldn't believe it when she weighed ten pounds, and Mary Catherine and Tom went running around finding things to weigh to make sure the scale was accurate. She measured 21½ inches long.

My placenta seemed like it was detaching very, very slowly, but it still hadn't come out by midday. I posted a question about it on a childbirth thread at mothering.com. Everything else was perfect—my uterus was shrinking, I wasn't bleeding a lot, the baby was nursing a ton—and I felt like I was just missing some little piece of knowledge that would help me out, but

I didn't feel like there was anything "wrong." A midwife who posts to the thread a lot offered me her cell phone number and I called when it had been 24 hours. She told me I could sort of twirl the placenta around to make the membranes rope up, and then reach up inside and gently wiggle them back and forth until they released. I got off the phone and did this and it was out in about 5 minutes. I took some pictures and put it in the freezer to plant in the spring.

Phoebe's Birth Story
Kelly Silliman

I think I had a couple contractions that may or may not have woken me up around 1 a.m. I got up to pee, and when I came back to bed, I woke Tom up to tell him I thought things might be starting but that we should definitely try to get some more rest. Tom started feeling nauseated, which he does when women go into labor, and so he got up to go to the bathroom, and while he was gone I had several more contractions. They felt mild, although they seemed to hurt more because my abdominal muscles were sore from coughing for three days. By the time Tom came back from the bathroom, he was feeling better but unsettled, and I was starting to have to breathe through the contractions.

After a couple minutes, I realized I wanted to be out of the bedroom, because I wasn't ready to wake up the kids and I was starting to want to vocalize a bit. The contractions kept coming and getting stronger, and my lower abdomen and lower back were hurting a lot. I suddenly realized I wanted to be in water. I have never felt drawn to water-birth personally, so this surprised me. I had Tom fill the bathtub, and there wasn't enough hot water, so he started boiling water on the stove. I got in and it felt so much better, except that the only way to have water covering my belly was to sit in it, which wasn't the best position for laboring though the contractions.

I remember sitting in the tub and looking at Tom and saying really calmly, "I don't want to do this anymore." I was thinking that it hurt so much, but that I was way too calm to be anywhere near actually birthing. I was listening to the noises I was making and they were so much less intense than when I birthed Arissa, so I figured I had a ways to go.

At some point I suddenly wanted out of the tub, so Tom helped me out and I went into the living room to be in front of the fire. I decided to lie down on the couch to try and relax through some contractions, which were getting longer and more intense, but certainly not on top of each other.

I started feeling like I had to pee, and told Tom I wanted to go to the bathroom. When I got up, though, I realized I was feeling pushy, and as I got down on hands and knees for the next contraction, my water broke. It was very dark, and I asked Tom to check it out because I was pretty sure it was full of meconium. When he confirmed that it was, I remember thinking really calmly that the baby needed to come out quickly. My body started pushing, and I could feel the head coming down and I yelled "Get the kids!"

The head started crowning and I squatted, trying to apply pressure to my perineum. It seemed to me to be taking a while (like five or ten minutes, but later when we looked at the time-stamps on the photos, we realized I only pushed for two minutes), and the head felt different to me. I actually wondered for a second if it was breech. The baby's face was sideways as it came out, and the head felt bigger than either Rosalie's or Arissa's, although we never measured, so I don't know. I also felt more stretching and "ring of fire" pain than before. I could feel the baby wiggling just before the body came out. I caught the body as it slid out, and laid her on the ground to remove the cord from around the back of the neck, and looked to see what gender we had. It was a girl!

I picked her up and held her. She was covered in meconium and vernix, but otherwise her color looked great and she was breathing and looked perfect. I think Rosalie had been watching the whole time; Arissa had been pretty sleepy, but when she heard the baby make noise she jumped up and came running over with a smile. It was just after 3 a.m.

My placenta came out around 4:20 a.m. It looked great, and Rosalie and Tom cut the cord. I'm not much of a bleeder, but there was still blood and meconium all over me and the baby that was drying, so we took a quick bath.

I am amazed each time I birth at how magical and routine it is at the same time. Each birth feels more a part of normal, everyday life, and I love being in the comfort of my own home with only my loved ones around me. It seems like such a perfect welcome to the world.

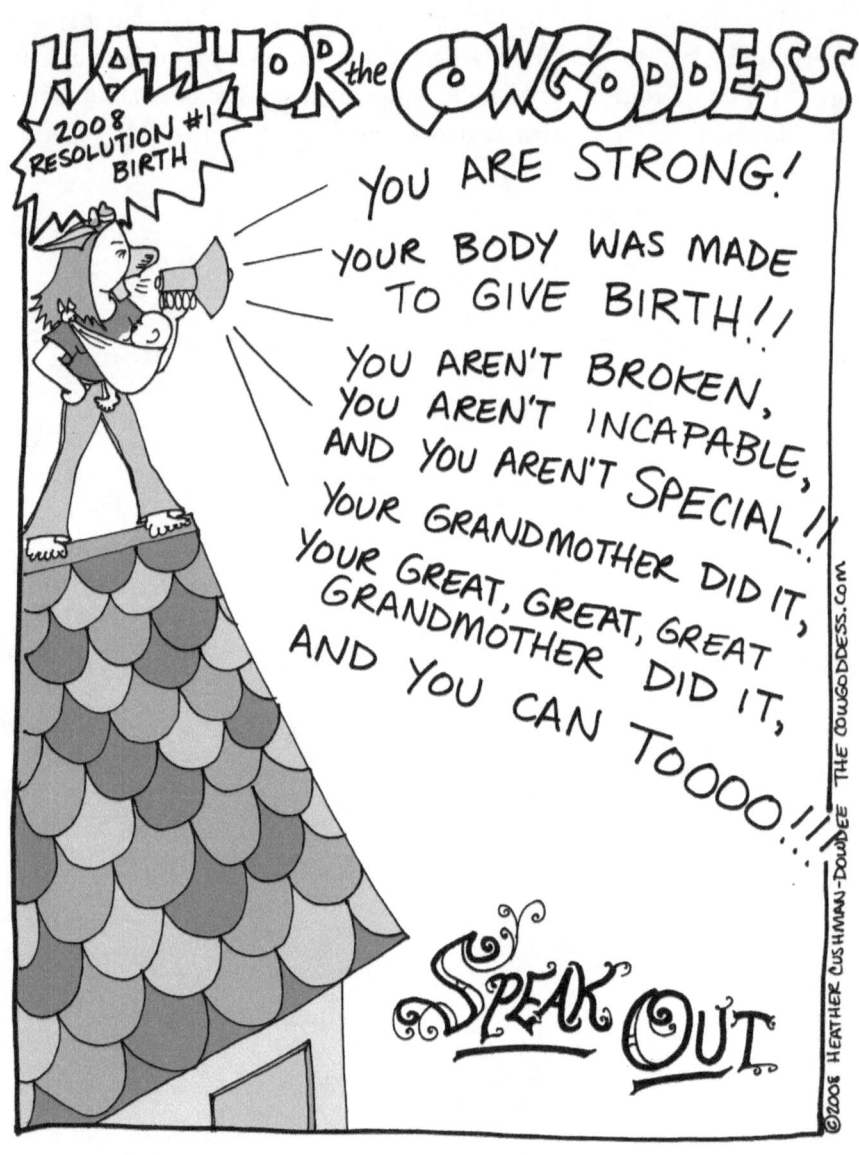

The Birth of Zoe Fae Mirick
Tasha Rose-Mirick

We fell to sleep around 1:30 a.m. At 3 I awoke with diarrhea pains so I went to the bathroom. Afterward I decided I was in too much pain to go back to bed and thought that I might *really* be in baby-producing labor this time. I told Rob I was going downstairs and he diligently followed, carting pillows with him.

Once we got downstairs it seems instinct took over and I began nesting. I lit a candle, the candle we lit on our wedding/handfasting day, and made ready the couch and the floor with a drop sheet and chux pads. I was having more and painful (in my hips only) contractions and I needed Rob more and more. I was not comfortable if he was very far from me.

I heard Grace wake up upstairs so I carted myself back up there and helped her to go potty. I contemplated keeping her up, but then decided against it as I didn't think the baby would come before Grace's normal waking time. I kissed Grace and tucked her back in telling her that the baby would be here soon. She was excited but fell back to sleep anyhow. I went back downstairs. Rob was camping out on the floor of the living room and I knelt down beside him. I tried to sit lotus to meditate through my contractions but it wasn't comfortable at all, so I got back onto my knees and leaned on Rob through a few more contractions before deciding that maybe the shower would feel nice and allow me to meditate a little. Rob made his nap spot on the bathroom floor in front of the washer and dryer while I got into the shower.

It was about 4:30 at this point and I stayed in the shower for about twenty-five minutes. It felt so wonderful but I started to feel like I had to eliminate again so I got out of the shower and toweled off. I sat down on the stool and had a very powerful contraction. I yelled to Rob, who was getting a watch to time contractions, that I thought the baby was coming. He came back into the bathroom ready to time and as he was walking in I had a contraction that broke my water. I felt the pop and then the warm gush that went into the toilet. I reached down and felt our daughters head. I yelled again, though Rob was right there, that the baby's head was there. He put the watch down and knelt in front of me. I told him that I needed to push and so I did. She came out head first and posterior, just like we anticipated. I pushed one more consecutive push and out came her body into the hands of her father. It was the most intimate and loving experience I had had with Rob. It was five o'clock a.m. and there was magic and faerie dust all around and the world stood still. We tipped her over to let her do the work in clearing herself out. I rolled her onto her back and began rubbing in her vernix while Rob went to get a receiving blanket to keep her warm. She wailed with all her might and she looked like a little, wet, pissed-off Chinese man.

After we had her covered, I stayed on the stool while Rob went to go get the new big sister. Grace was tired and weary, but instantly in love with her baby sister. After a few minutes as a new family, we moved into the living room. I couldn't put Zoe onto my chest because the placenta was at the very top of my uterus, making the cord snug if I tried. I didn't want to accidentally rip out my placenta, so I stayed seated with her on my lap. I attempted to nurse her right away, but she was tired and not interested in eating, nor would she be for quite a while that day.

We initially planned on a lotus birth for Zoe, but soon it didn't feel like what was meant to be as my placenta was still inside two hours later. Rob cut the cord that bound her to me and about a half hour later I expelled my placenta. That deliverance was more work, it seemed, than giving birth to Zoe. The contractions were harder and actually induced pain, whereas the labor contractions didn't hurt so much, nor did pushing her out of my body.

118

The placenta fell out of me and into the toilet. I retrieved it and put it into the colander to drain so we could inspect it. It was beautiful. Grace was grossed out but intrigued at the same time to see the sac that her sister lived in for so long.

Our first day was long and tiring and amazing. We have a link to our home, to our universe and to each other like no one else can say. I am in love with my husband even more than I was before and it increases every day. This child is the completion of every dream I had when Rob and I were just teenagers in love so long ago. I sobbed later that night as we three laid in our bed together. I felt so much love that I thought I might just burst wide open. I fell to sleep with my lover and our child. I fell to sleep happier than I had ever been in my life.

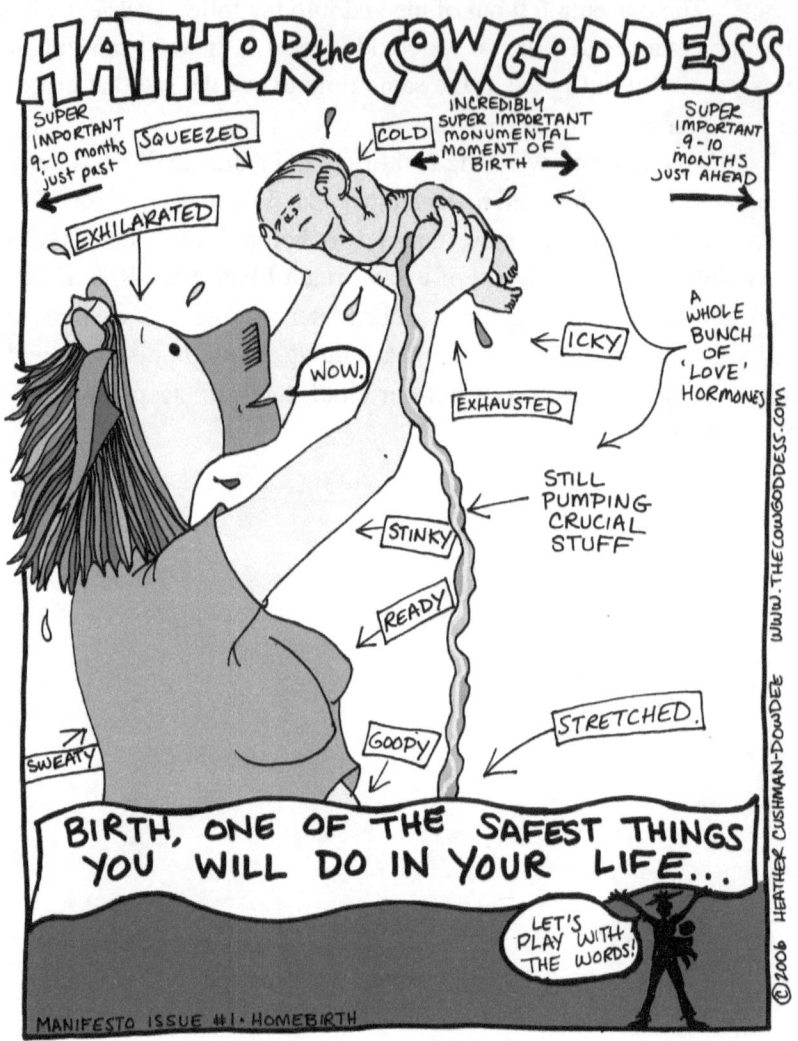

Squeaky's Birth Story
Valerie Wassergeburt

I woke up the morning of December 12, 2006, around 3:30 a.m. to contractions. It was uncomfortable lying down, so I moved to the recliner. The contractions were so much easier to handle when I was upright. It was cool in the house and I tried to cover up with a small blanket and Jon's jacket. I didn't want to wake him up by going into the bedroom to get another blanket. I was in a hazy sense of vague awareness since I was so sleepy and I tried to sleep, but they were coming pretty steadily so I moved to the toilet at 6 a.m. and then my yoga ball in the living room. I love the yoga ball! Being able to rock my hips around with cushy perineum support was heavenly and made everything manageable. I held onto the legs of a bar stool in front of me for support. At 7 a.m. Jon woke up and I asked him to fill up my inflatable tub and hook up the new hoses. I rocked on my birth ball and listened as each section of the tub was filled with air. The contractions were coming exactly five minutes apart. I'd relax in between them and then start rolling my hips in anticipation just before the five minutes ticked by on the wall clock. It felt good to change direction too, first rolling my hips to the right and then switching to counterclockwise circling during the contraction. That also gave me something to focus on as the contraction peaked and passed.

I told Jon I was ready to get in the tub. I was at four minutes apart (I never checked internally for dilation, somehow that just seems wrong to me —too intrusive. I feel sure it would have slowed or reversed my progress) and got online to check my favorite forum and read the advice the wise women had left me. I got in the tub when the contractions started coming at three minutes apart. The water reached the top of the bottom three inflatable rings. Time was flying by and I leaned over the edge of the tub for each contraction. I held the hot water hose aimed at my lower back, which felt very relaxing. The water really did help! I figured I had a long time yet as they hardly hurt. They felt like average menstrual cramps for a few seconds at the peak and then complete relief. They were very "intense" though and my face would sweat profusely during each. I covered my face with a towel to catch the sweat. During a few I'd bite at the tub or bite down on the towel. I fell asleep in between each; I remember strange but short dreams.

Being alone in the house was pure bliss, if only for just a few minutes. I felt free to really relax. I tried vocalizing but quickly realized that isn't for me. No, I was happiest to be alone, quiet, reflective and free. I feel I made a huge amount of progress then. Strong yet gentle contractions as my cervix completed opening. Not long after that I got the urge to push and the contractions felt really good. They felt like a huge relief, it was such a dramatic difference in the sensations!

I was surprised that I now felt like pushing—after all I hadn't even realized I was in transition. It was so peaceful! The day seemed to be going by quickly until this point. Pushing ... well, I pushed for more than three hours. I had read it is a good thing because it slowly stretches you and firstborns usually take longer anyway. I grunted with each push and noticed Jon looked worried that I was hurting, so I told him that the grunting was from the effort of pushing—it didn't hurt. His face brightened up. It was much like grunting with the effort of picking up a very heavy box. Interestingly, in this new pushing stage, I didn't mind being watched at all. The work of labor and birth now seemed more physical. I no longer needed to "go inward." Time, space...I was aware of it all. It was a completely new labor, it seemed. I was also blessed with a surge of newfound energy!

Finally around 3:30 I said enough is enough because I was so comfortable I thought maybe I was slowing my progress, and got out of the pool. I wiggled my hips and felt the baby move down. That was an amazing, wonderful feeling! The baby felt perfect and completely natural moving through my body. I had read about how some women experienced discomfort as they felt their pelvises moving apart for the baby. There was absolutely no discomfort for me, it just felt "right." Then I started waddling through the house squatting and grunting and laughing. I must have been a sight—wild wet hair in a falling down bun. It felt great pushing, but I was ready for Squeaky, as we had come to call the baby, to meet us. Jon said at one point I grabbed the stool and squatted down in front of Helen (my favorite hen, whose breed, Serama, is sensitive to cold so I brought her and her two newly hatched chicks inside to keep them all warm), and stared her in the eye and grunted real loud. I tried getting on the bed and pushing, but I didn't like that position and didn't feel it helped any. I got on the floor and kneeled on one knee and felt Squeaky crown and the soft hairy head.

I waddled back to the bathroom and held a small mirror under me and gently opened my vagina with my fingers and saw his head with wet, dark hair! What an empowering moment! Very encouraged, I returned to the bedroom and got back in the pool and kneeled and pushed. Switched to all fours and pushed with every ounce of strength I had, roaring like a lion. I felt this huge bulge, aimed at my tailbone. I roared and pushed and then burning…pushed, even more burning. This was the first time I'd say the birth hurt, but I was doing it!!! (In retrospect, perhaps I could have been a bit more patient and allowed myself to stretch slower, but it seemed I had waited so long already!)

I took a quick breath in between pushes so Squeaky wouldn't slip back. My baby was almost here so I dismissed the pain and pushed, the burn, and then out came the head! I called out for Jon to come in and join me; the baby was being born. We were soooooooo thrilled! He got down on the floor behind me and said the cord was around the neck, and that it was loose so he slipped it over the baby's head. I pushed and wiggled and the shoulders came out and Jon said they were folded towards each other and touching. Of all things I had a hard time with the hips. I looked behind me and saw the little body half out of me, floating in the water, gray and amazing.

I pushed really hard and tried subtle changes in position, and I think it was because the baby was angled upwards from floating in the water. I asked Jon to angle baby downwards. It started kicking inside of me then, which didn't feel good, and I said, "Ouch! Stop that!" because I thought it was something Jon was doing, and then the baby came out. Jon lifted him out of the water and announced, "It's a boy!!" and I laughed, "Well, of course!" It was 4:30 p.m.. We had our Nathan Forrest in our arms! We had picked out that name for him years and years before he was even conceived, back when we were just dating!

Jon handed Nathan to me and I sat back against the soft inflatable wall of the birth pool. We draped a small blanket over him and then Jon turned the hot water hose back on to warm the water some more. Nathan opened his eyes and quietly looked around as we ooh'ed and ahh'ed over him and rubbed him as he took his first breaths of air and turned pink. I gently massaged his vernix-covered skin in complete amazement and inspected the tiny hands and feet and counted fingers and toes. He looked perfect and beautiful. Jon got the camera then and took some pictures. Nathan already showed interest in nursing! His dark eyes scanned what they could and finally settled on my bare chest. He knew just what to do! We were very impressed. Jon said, "You might not have had time to read the book yet (I was intending to read my breastfeeding books in the next two weeks as I spent most of my reading time during the last nine months concentrating on birthing), but he knows what to do!" Jon put a new shower curtain on the bed and covered it with towels and I tried sitting there for a bit but it was rather uncomfortable. The umbilical cord was short, just long enough to get the baby up to my chest. I was completely worn out. Jon helped me adjust around on the bed trying to get comfortable by placing multiple pillows behind me but then helped me back off the bed.

We cut the cord an hour and a half later; it was all white and cold by now. We laid him in the top drawer of the dresser and Jon put on the clamps and sliced the umbilical cord in two with a sterile razor blade and took him in his arms. I felt a pang in my heart as I realized we were now two completely separate people, suddenly feeling a bit empty and alone. Jon held him while I took a shower. I was surprised how hard I had to push to get the placenta out...for some reason I was under the impression it would just slither out easily. It was 7 p.m. when I squatted down over a Tupperware bowl and pushed really hard and it finally came out and plopped right into the bowl, fully intact, thick and beautiful. I victoriously called out that I got it out and grabbed my camera and took a picture of it. Jon was sitting on the couch with Nathan then and I showed it to him. Then I cut a sliver off and put it under my tongue for about five minutes before swallowing it. It wasn't bad, reminiscent of steak. Haha. It is supposed to help lessen bleeding since it is full of hormones and also lessens the chance of postpartum depression. I put the cover on the Tupperware and put the placenta in the freezer to plant under Nathan's tree later.

I called my mom at 7:30; I don't think I've ever heard her so excited. He weighed in at 6 pounds and 13 ounces and was 20 inches long.

Soooooooooooooooooooooo cute.

A Family Freebirth
Kelli Lincoln

My water broke at 3 p.m., as I was heating something up on the stove and dancing with the kids to "Rock Lobster" by the B-52s. Not really dancing, but just bouncing, which apparently was enough to open things up! I felt a little trickle, raised a brow and went to the bathroom. As soon as I sat down on the toilet, there was a huge gush of water. I had always wondered what it felt like to start labor this way, since my with my other two births the sack didn't break till the end, and I had been in water at the time, so I didn't feel anything, really. So I was fascinated by how much water was in there! I must have returned to the toilet about six times, each with a similar gush of water. At 3:15, I lost my plug, which was also different from before. I had bloody show and stringy mucous with my first two, but not an actual *plug*—well this time, there was really a plug! It looked and felt like a clear marshmallow, same shape and everything — totally cool! I wasn't really in labor, with contractions irregular and pretty light, as they had been for weeks, so I felt like it could be hours or maybe days before the birth, and felt I should rest.

At 1:11 a.m., the baby woke me with a big kick which was followed by a doozy of a contraction. I had been having them all along, but this one convinced me it was time to get up. So I woke Abe, and we went out to the dining room, where we basically sat and looked at one another between contractions while we enjoyed the warmth of the wood stove. The contractions were definitely heating up, but it's just so hard to know where you are on that labor continuum at this stage. I was leaning on the kitchen counter during contractions at this point, with Abe behind me supporting me. I would press up against him, almost sitting on his lap (although we were standing), and I remember that his warmth and strength were so soothing and necessary. I felt the baby move at one point and was happy to know that all was well in there.

Contractions were about every two-to-three minutes at this point, but they were only about twenty seconds long, until one big one-minute long-one, during which I felt the baby slip down a bit. From then, the contractions really picked up, I felt that first involuntary push, and I was starting to vocalize more. Abe was still holding me from behind, and I remember his voice soft and low in my ear, reminding me to keep my sounds low, and he vocalized with me to help me focus.

At 3:45 (Abe scribbled notes of things I said all night, which is the only reason I know the timing of these things), I had the slightest twinges of nausea, and I remember saying quite calmly that I was in transition. Fifteen minutes later, the involuntary and very real pushing had taken over, which was sort of a relief. I mean, this is the part that really hurts, but for some reason there is a part of my brain that really enjoys it, and I've felt the same for each of my three births. We had moved to the bedroom, because I had been having a hard time getting into a position that felt just right. I remember pushing on my lower belly during the contractions, trying to help push that baby's body under or around my pelvis—it just felt like it was in the way, and I sort of even wanted to lay down, but I didn't.

This baby was coming! I wanted to feel the head, and I was a little surprised at how large it seemed. I clearly remember how Thane's head felt in the palm of my hand at this point, and this head barely even FIT in my hand! I also expected the head to be followed by a large gush of slippery little body, since that's what I experienced both times before, but instead, there was quite a pause. Quite an uncomfortable pause! Abe saw something near the neck, and put a finger there to see if it was the cord, but it was a hand instead! Another contraction and the hands and shoulders emerged, but dang if there wasn't another pause! Abe asked if he should do something and I wanted to tell him to pull the baby *out*—because ouch, I tell you, being stretched that far for that long!!—but I didn't say anything, since he probably would have, and I knew I didn't really want him to pull on the baby. One last contraction brought the rest of the baby out into Abe's hands, a gift we had made together last spring finally making its entrance into our family, surrounded in love *by* that family. Truly beautiful. (It was 4:26 a.m., so active labor was about three hours.)

Abe laid the baby on the bed next to me, and he appeared to be asleep! The cord was fairly short, so I didn't bring him up to me, but just rubbed him all over, trying to catch my breath. After a minute or two of rubbing the baby, he opened his eyes with a little squeak and just looked around, totally alert, not crying or anything. Just sort of curious about this new, colder, brighter, room.

About thirty minutes after the baby's birth, I felt a few more contractions and the urge to squat up and push out that placenta. It seemed huge to me, like another whole baby. We put it in the placenta bowl (we've used it for each birth!) and I sat up a bit to see if Emrys wanted to nurse. He did nurse for a few minutes, and then we all five fell asleep for about two and a half hours. When we woke up, Rhanna cut the cord (it felt so very cold!) I looked at the placenta thoroughly at that point, and it was huge, and just beautiful. Perfectly formed, intact, and. . .well, luscious. I felt a wave of thanks toward it, for helping me grow a perfect baby.

Our Journey of Trust
Rebekah Costello

Thursday morning, April 19th, 2007: I was startled out of the deepest sleep I'd had in a week at 3:30 a.m. with a contraction I was already on my hands and knees moaning through before really waking up. "Ooooooooohhh, baby, baby, baby, baby!" So much pressure down below it was phenomenal. When it was over, I just laid back down and went to sleep. I never really even opened my eyes. I remember thinking that it wasn't fair to do this to me while I was sleeping when it wasn't going to happen for another month, anyway. Sometime later I came awake to another contraction that had me up and moving around the bed, panting and moaning. Went right back to sleep. My attitude at this point was, "Whatever, body, cry wolf as much as you like, I don't even care, I'm sleeping, thankyouverymuch!" I didn't watch the clock per se, didn't time contractions, but occasionally I'd look to see what time it was because I *refused* to get out of bed until it was closer to time to get up. I'd really spent enough nights getting *no sleep* so I was going to sleep between contractions for as long as I could stand it. But around 6:30 they were making it impossible to do so. I decided to get in the shower because I figured they would let up around 7:30 anyway and I really, really wanted to sleep. So a hot shower would probably just facilitated the "drop back" of contractions and then maybe I'd get another hour to *sleep*

The shower did nothing, if anything I just felt pukey in the hot water so I got out and went potty. Oh, wow, look at that, bloody show. I mean, I hadn't had any for two days and now it was bright red and copious. Before it was bloody mucous now it was mucous-y blood. The contraction I had on the toilet was hard and I believe I was moaning through that one, too. I went downstairs to do my morning thing, still telling myself it was going to go away. I figured I'd update my livejournal and lay down on the couch so as not to disturb my husband and then they'd let up again...like they had every other morning this week. I didn't want to believe I was in active labor, I just wanted to sleep. By 8 a.m., though, I knew that I didn't *care* if I was in active labor or not, I could not possibly cope with those contractions all day, again, by myself with my daughter. No way, Jose! I went upstairs to find out if Paul would stay home with me. The thought of having to care for my daughter with contractions that were so hard I couldn't talk through them was just overwhelming and had me in tears. I asked Paul what it would take to get him to stay home today. He asked me why I wanted him to do that (he wasn't really awake yet) and of course, I started to have a contraction right then so I sort of gritted out, between my teeth, "Why do you *think*!?!??!" He said, "You think you're in labor?" and I said, "I honestly don't know but I *do* know that I cannot do this by myself today, I just can't."

I was still thinking it might peter out and that I'd be pretty upset if it did because these contractions *hurt*. I mean, there was pre-labor ouchies and then there was *oh my god the pressure the pressure give me counter-pressure now* ouchies. See the difference?

I couldn't stand the tub (Fat woman + uncomfortable bathtub + intense back labor = crap). I got out. I put my pajamas back on and went downstairs and continued for a while, laboring on my knees, my chest draped onto the couch. I'd start making noise through a contraction and Paul would rush into the living room, from the kitchen, and give me counter-pressure and rub my back and talk to me through them (I still chuckle at the mental picture of my husband rushing through the house with a towel over one shoulder and a spatula in one hand, to give me counter-pressure). When he left the room, at one point, Elizabeth climbed up on my back (like she was going to "ride the horsey") and just her sitting in the exact right spot helped immensely. She then leaned forward and draped herself across my whole back and said, "Daddy's coming, Mama, Daddy's coming, it's all right." I laughed a lot between contractions while she was with me. Oh, I'm so blessed.

The contractions got closer and closer together. They didn't seem to have any real pattern to them really, at first, except I would get them in clusters. One, two, three, a break...one, two, three, etc. I had this intense pressure in my vagina with every contraction and it would wrap up the bottom of my uterus and into the small of my back with this incredible pressure. The pain was all down below, too, just in the bottom half. The pain in back was just immense and oftentimes it was the only thing I could think of. I was afraid of the pain!! I was, I was terrified of it and that in and of itself was a shock because I had not previously been afraid of labor pain. In retrospect, I believe there are three reasons for this: One was simply that I was just plain tired! I'd been laboring for a week! The second was that I subconsciously feared that they would get even worse because my only point of reference was the pitocen-induced labor I experienced while birthing Elizabeth. The third reason is that the shock of having a baby much earlier than I anticipated left me rigid. I was just blindsided by the reality that I really *was* having this baby a month early. I was so incredibly tense that Paul noticed and he started to talk me down. "You can do this, you're doing an incredible job, Babe, you need to relax, don't fight it, you can do it," just a litany with every contraction. His talking worked, before I hit transition I was able to do something I couldn't do at all with Elizabeth's labor. I stopped shouting through contractions and instead breathed through them.

When I look back on this labor, I remember this time as being the most peaceful. Paul was sitting on the couch, I was on my knees in front of him, leaning into his lap and I had my arms wrapped around his waist. He had his hands on my back and his head by my ear and with every contraction he just talked to me softly and I concentrated on expanding my belly around the immense sensations there. I cannot say I felt no pain, because I can't perceive of that feeling any other way, really. But I felt so much more than the pain. It was a fight, it really was, to stay on top of that pain and experience the rest of it but it was *bliss*. I can't explain it. It hurt like a *beotch*, no doubt about it, but it was *so much more*. I would feel a contraction building and would expand my belly around it, like we were in competition with each other, my outer layers with my inner. Or maybe more like we were dancing. It was like: my baby, covered by my womb, covered by my belly, covered by my husband, covered by Yahweh. In my mind, womb would pull and clamp and my belly would expand and expand over it like I was trying to draw that painful feeling *outward* instead of losing myself *in* it. I would take these huge, slow breaths and fallow myself to open wider and wider and to not clench anything but my hands on Paul's arms or his shirt. That part was awesome.

I don't know how long that lasted but at some point transition started because I just started to get angry with every contraction. I felt like labor was progressing too fast and not quickly enough. This wasn't supposed to be happening right now, I was supposed to have another few weeks to prepare. Contractions were supposed to stop again, like before, so I could sleep and just *who was it* that declared I should get a week of minimal sleep before doing this? Oh I was angry, I was exhausted, I was afraid. Every feeling of letdown, of anger, built-up tension and every feeling of sorrow from the last several months just came pouring out of me. I don't remember all of what I said. Mostly a barrage of "I don't want to do this anymore" and "I can't" and *"I need a break!!!"* I could not have articulated anything else coherently if I tried. I started sobbing. I've never cried so hard in my life. So much intense energy was flowing through me and I just could not contain it all. I couldn't integrate the pain and the energy and the intense emotions. Nope. Mouth gets free rein, my heart is open and my mind was just bubbling over.

Transition ended as suddenly as it started. I had a contraction that was very different. Pain in my back took a back burner to the *downward* feeling contraction (I was standing through most of transition and I had my arms around Paul's neck). I really just like, squatted down into this contraction and just *"Oh my God"* through it. My whole body shook with the force of it. I felt like it was pushy except it felt very strange. The third one of these ended with me giving a test push and my water breaking on the feet of everyone standing around me. At this point, Paul said, "Oh, thank you so much for not puking on my feet, which is what I thought you were doing just now!" Laughter, all around. That sound will stay with me forever, I think.

I realized that the contractions had just stopped and suddenly, I was okay. No more whirlwind of thoughts, emotions, and feelings flooding me. I said, "Oh good, a break!" and sat down on the couch. I was okay, I was in this little place of waiting in my head and felt like everything was on hold for a minute. I know there was conversation and I know I participated in it but I really am not sure what was said. All of a sudden, I just needed to stand back up. So I did. And then I had another contraction or two and then another one that was *huge*. Then, like in a dream I had at the beginning of this pregnancy,

I felt the whole baby come down in one huge, sliding motion and slam into my perineum. I wanted to push but something told me to wait and see what was presenting. I gave a test push and then said, "What *is* that?" *What is it????* Paul came back in and got down and took a peek. Paul said: "It's a head, *Oh, wait*, that's a foot and a butt!!" Then, I felt a squirm and two feet kicked their way out of me and into the air, of their own volition! This baby wanted to come *out*. A contraction and a biiiig puuush. Oh, that felt good, it was the best push *ever*. Baby out to her umbilicus. I heard someone say, "Oh, it's so small!" Mixed feelings with that announcement. A brief brush of fear which I shoved out of my mind as quickly as it entered with a fierce determination that everything would be fine. As I was doing that, the baby kicked her daddy's hands. I remembered another dream from over a year ago of me having a baby breech and I just laughed out loud. I couldn't believe it!!

Well, I wasn't having contractions again. So I pushed without one just to see what would happen. Nothing, nothing happened at all. She didn't budge. So I tried again, this time squatting into it a bit. That felt wrong. So I turned around and leaned over the couch again and tried again. Nothing, not so much as a smidgen of a budge. I prayed out loud, "Abbah, I know this is you, I know this is okay, what am I missing? I trust you, tell me!" She punched my in the birth canal and like a light bulb, duh, her arms!!! "Hey, where are her arms?" Several voices at once, "They are still inside." "Okay, honey, reach up in there and bring her arms down." He started to poke around like he was afraid he'd hurt me. "Don't worry about hurting me *just do it!*" He said, "Okay, Babe," and poked two fingers in there and hooked an arm and brought it down. He told me her other arm came down on its own. *Then* I had a contraction and pushed the rest of her out in one push. My legs were shaking so badly at this point that all I could do for a second was breathe deeply with my face in the couch cushion. Everyone was so quiet I realized that I needed to turn around and tend to the baby.

I could tell from the hush in the room that everyone was worried. I just smiled to myself. I knew everything was okay, despite that nagging little snarky voice in the back of my head that said, "What if..what if...what if..." I thrust it away and turned around and sat down on the edge of the couch, on a Chux pad, and Paul handed me our daughter. She was seemingly quite limp and that purplish color that babies who are pinking up turn. It was hard to see through all the vernix. Paul looked right into my eyes in that moment and I couldn't read his expression, it was just too full of too many things. I took my daughter in my arms and put her face down over my left arm and started talking to her. "Abigail, come on baby, I love you!" I started to rub and gently pat her back, making sure her head was at a slight incline towards the floor. She moved her foot and I noticed she was getting pinker by the second. I could feel the cord pulsing between us. I had a fleeting thought to call an ambulance but brushed it aside gently, to be considered later if it was needed. I kept talking, kept rubbing and she squeaked, coughed, and squeaked again. I turned her over without really thinking about it and sucked her mouth out, spat, sucked her nose out, spat, nose twice more and by the time I was finished with that she was hollering about it to the whole world. Eyes open, lungs going, lip trembling. "I'm *here,* already, goodness, just don't do *that* again!" We wrapped her up with a blanket, a hat came from somewhere and everyone was smiling. Welcome, Abigail!!

We waited about an hour to cut the cord. It was totally limp and we clamped it on baby-side and didn't bother with my side as I'd delivered it maybe fifteen minutes after Abby was born. She was *tiny* (she weighed 4 pounds, 10 ounces and was 17 3/4 inches long). I could tell she was good by the time she'd stopped crying, there was no gurgle left to her breathing and she was just looking around with her little hands folded like she was surveying her surroundings sort of grumpily. She was perfect. She looked like a wizened old lady, and that made me laugh. I tried to nurse her but she wasn't at all interested in that, so skin-to-skin for a while and then I passed her off to Paul so I could get cleaned up. I went up, took a bath and carefully checked around for tears or lacerations. Nothing. Not so much as a skid mark (that I could feel). I came back downstairs after getting dressed to discover the entire mess was cleaned up. Paul said it took about five minutes (he just rolled it all up in the aforementioned plastic mat and threw it in the trash). I settled onto the couch with my new baby girl and offered her a chance to nurse. This time she was ready and opened right up and we began that "eyeball talk" that all mothers have with their babies. I was just enthralled. I couldn't believe how tiny she was, how perfect every little detail was. I still feel that way, looking at her is like looking at a tiny little miracle.

The Birth Story of Gwyneth Kai

At 12:30 a.m. on June 29 (twenty-three days past my due date) I heard a *pop!* Then a gurgle and then a *splash* and water poured out from between my legs! I half yelled "Kevin, my water broke!" (Quiet, don't wake the kiddies) He looked at me *huh*? And then jumped out of bed and ran into the kitchen or "the birthing room" as we imagined it and started moving the table and chairs out to make room for the pool. I, meanwhile, am floundering on the bed with torrents of water gushing out of me. And you know what I'm thinking? I'm remembering that I am on the mattress *without* a mattress pad. Kevin finally comes to the room and sticks his head in to see if I need anything...yes, a towel would be nice. While he sets up the birth pool I stand in the bathtub for a few minutes, then I sit on the toilet and have the first contraction, then two more about two minutes apart, then a doozy that makes me think that the bath-mat looks really comfortable. So the next time Kevin sticks his head in the door I am lying on the bathroom floor. I decide soon after that contraction that in actuality the bath-mat is a very uncomfortable place, so I head into the kitchen.

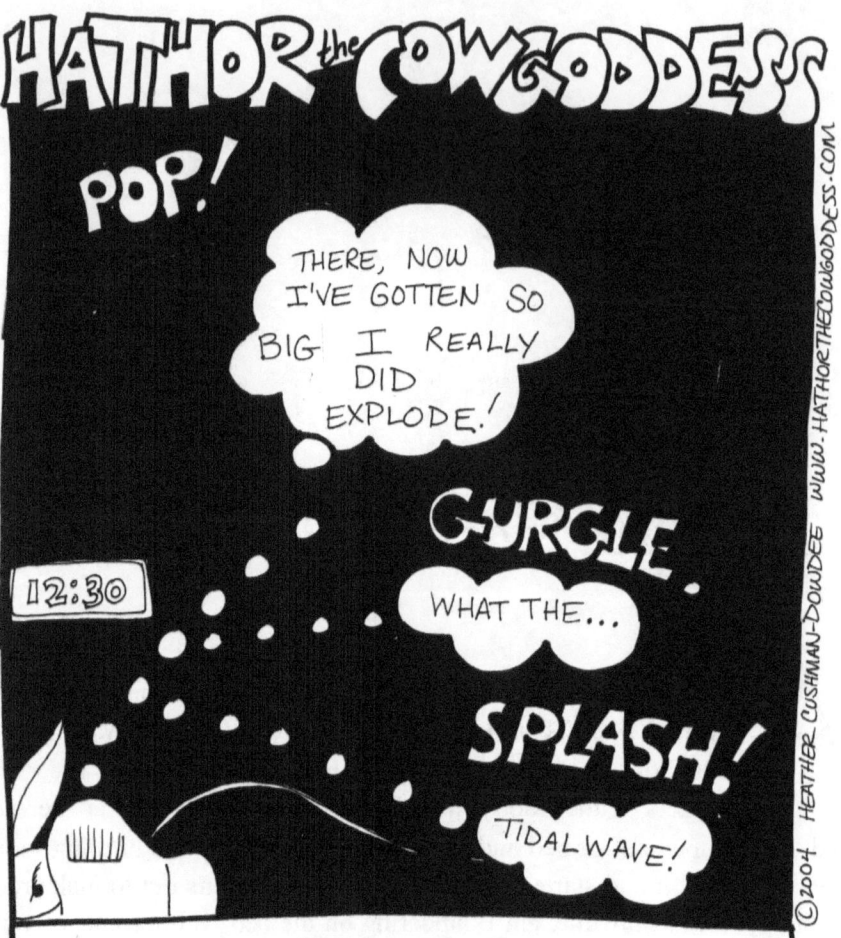

"BANG !!!???***!!!

PIGLET LAY THERE, WONDERING WHAT HAD HAPPENED. AT FIRST HE THOUGHT THAT THE WHOLE WORLD HAD BLOWN UP; AND THEN HE THOUGHT THAT ONLY THE FOREST PART OF IT HAD; AND THEN HE THOUGHT THAT PERHAPS ONLY HE HAD, AND HE WAS NOW ALONE ON THE MOON OR SOMEWHERE..."

— A.A. MILNE

I announce that I am really hungry, but Kevin talks me into a glass of water and we chat for a minute about what a crazy feeling that was to have my water break like that out of nowhere! Then I got into the birth pool. It was full about a quarter of the way and I told Kevin to stop filling because I wanted to be able to add warm water as it cooled and I was sure my labor was going to be many more hours.

I sat in the water through about eight contractions that were fairly easy. Then I thought I was going to throw up, but assured Kevin that the desire to hurl cookies was completely normal. He gave me a pot. I allowed this sign of impending transition to pass without notice because I was so sure that I still had hours left. I had a couple more contractions that I vocalized through. Kind of like a moose singing: *ooooooh hoooooow ooooow oooh* like that. Kevin asked if I should get out of the pool and move about a bit which seemed like a good idea.

I made it into a chair that was right by the pool in time for two contractions on top of each other that got me really howling. Kevin wiped off my face because it was incredibly hot in that kitchen what with the giant pool of really hot water and all the windows being closed (we live in a seven hundred and fifty square foot apartment with neighbors all around and it was the middle of summer). I asked for something to drink and experienced the laboring phenomena I had heard of, where you are holding a cup and you can't get it to your mouth. I'm staring at it and cannot bring it closer! I want to drink, but my arm will not cooperate! I now realize why bendy straws are included in every birth kit, unfortunately there was no time to get one out of the box.

I asked Kevin to set up a nest by the couch, still determined to move around to help the baby come, without realizing the birth was imminent! While he was arranging things I had a couple of massive contractions, and then he helped me to the living room "birth annex." We paused for another doozy of a contraction, and I'm beginning to think that I don't have the capability to withstand much more of this, but am still sure that I have two more hours at least…

I sit on my knees by the couch and have a contraction that lifts my body into the air and feels almost like I'm pushing! Okay, now so as not to spoil the goddess-like miracle of birth I'm going to add in brackets (so that you can skip over this part if you have a weak stomach) a part of the birth story that was very unpleasant for me [and I'm pooping!] My litany of phrases during the contraction totally changed from the moose like stuff from before to Oh no Oh NO Oh NO [oh shit, oh shit, oh shit because of the poop] and then Oh oh oh oh oh and stuff like that. I have two of those before we decide to go back to the pool.

Just in time for another one, Oh no Oh no Oh no [oh shit oh shit oh shit because I'm pooping again, how much could there possibly be? I'm thinking that I've been with this man for seventeen years and he's never had to wipe my butt before.] I am facing the birth pool wall on my knees and lifting up with the contractions. There is a pause. Then another contraction in which I am totally bearing down. Unmistakably. [And of course I'm pooping again. It crosses my mind to go sit on the toilet, but for the first time I actually think I may be close to having a baby!] As soon as that contraction stops I tell Kevin that I'm pushing. I don't know if this was news to him or not, but he got into the pool [which is impressive considering that there is… um, poop in there]. The next contraction I put my fingers inside myself to check and I feel a little lump which is decidedly foreign, could it be head? I tell Kevin the baby is coming! Another contraction and then Kevin tells me that he can feel the head too. The next contraction my vagina starts to burn so I add that to my litany too, oh no oh no oh o [oh shit oh shit oh shit, I'm not pooping anymore but I still want to say it for some reason] and then owy ow ow it burns oh ow oh no like that. Another one and more of the head and then *head*! Kevin announces it, but I already knew, I ask which way it's facing (for some reason this late in the game I still need to know the baby's position.) Kevin says its facing him. I feel Relief. I tell Kevin not to worry, this is the lull, and during the next contraction the shoulders will come. But there was one more with no change, and then I said, "Don't pull!" and Kevin said, "I'm not pulling!" so I knew that the baby was turning and *voila*! I felt a little body squirm around inside of me and then with a push, out slid Gwyneth. Kevin caught and then I turned around and he put her right into my lap, pale and still for about a second and then a little cough splutter and then a hearty cry! Yes!

It was 3 a.m.

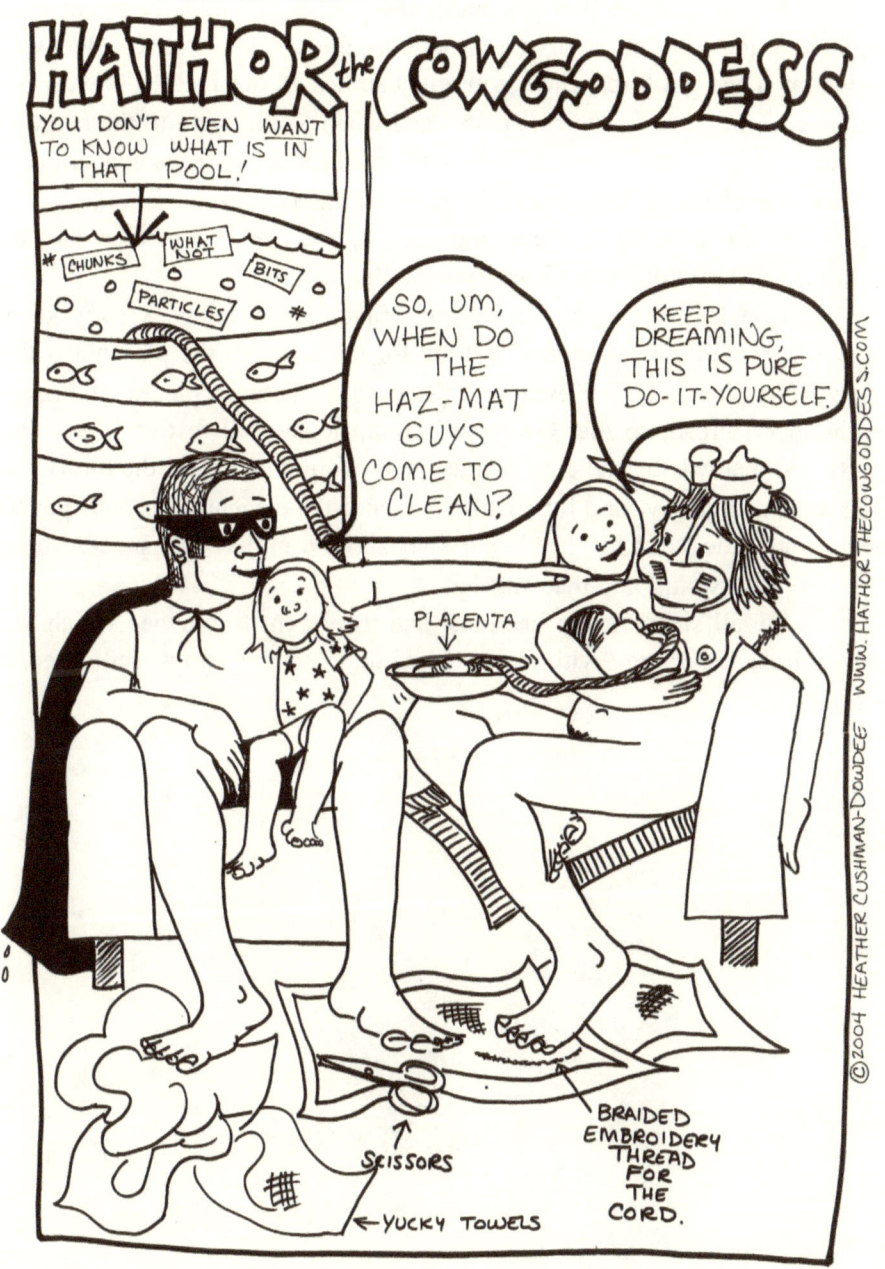

We decided we best get out of the pool which quickly became less miracle water and more of a cesspool as the minutes passed. We were exhilarated and goofy-psyched, with giant smiles on our faces. I moved over to the couch nest in the "birth annex" and when Kevin went to the bedroom to get more blankets for Gwyneth he saw my eldest daughter Isobel sitting up in bed. She claims to have heard the baby crying. (I want to remind you that our apartment is seven hundred and fifty square feet and neither daughter heard me carrying on! What is up with that?)

Isobel came to pay her respects first, then went back to wake up Fiona, they all gathered around in time for me to expel the placenta with a lovely plooping sound. Kevin tied the cord with three pieces of braided embroidery thread, so that Gwyneth's stump looked all festive like a little party and then we cut the cord (about forty-five minutes after the birth). She had remained gurgly for a little while, but once the placenta was out I put her feet a bit higher than her head, and after about a minute she sneezed out a bunch of snotty stuff and that was that.

We all shared a big breakfast and then went to our bed which was now a little less roomy with our new addition and fell into a well-deserved sleep.

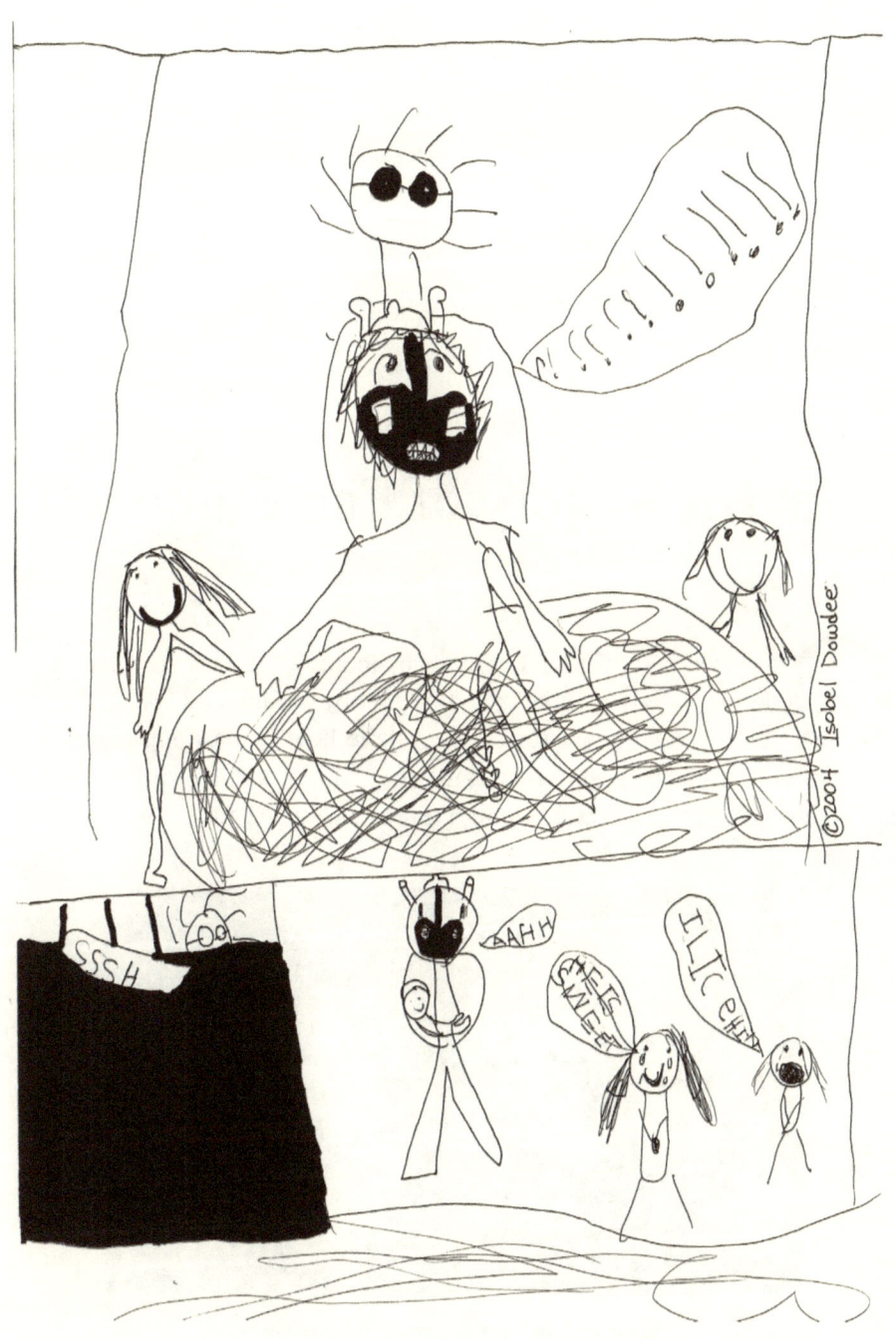

The Birth Story of Ean Campbell

O n March 31, 2009, I woke up about 3:15 a.m. to what were definitely contractions. Kind of crampy feeling and low, under the tummy. I lay there for the next three hours with a big goofy grin on my face because first of all, this is *labor* and it's still three days before my due date and second of all, these are *easy* and I can't wait to meet the baby.

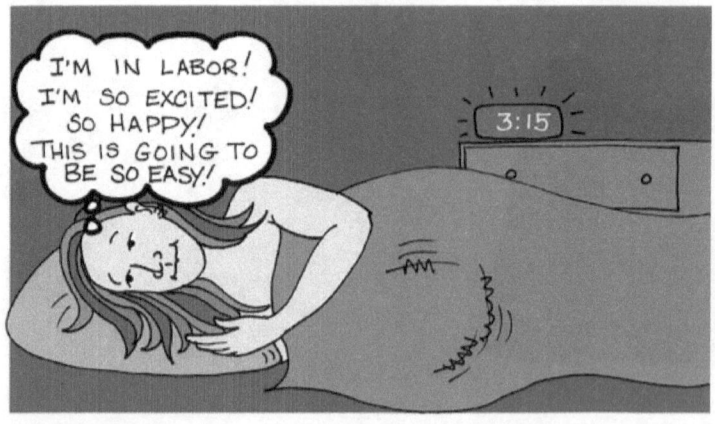

Then the contractions all but stop when I get up.

I went to the grocery store with the kids, which was an exciting experience (what if my water breaks?) and I still have that goofy grin on my face. "I'm in labor! and nobody knows!"

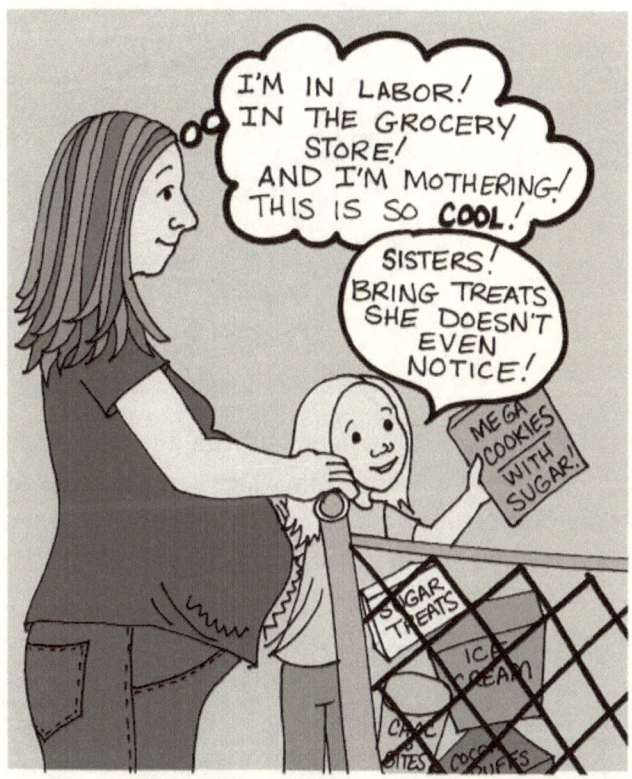

At about 3 p.m. I decided that the contractions were becoming difficult enough to climb into the bathtub. Of course my littlest had to climb in with me. Which is how my husband found us at about 3:45. I officially declared myself "in labor" and we had to talk that through for a second because I am always late, and this was early, and what do I mean I'm in labor, and could I be mistaken?

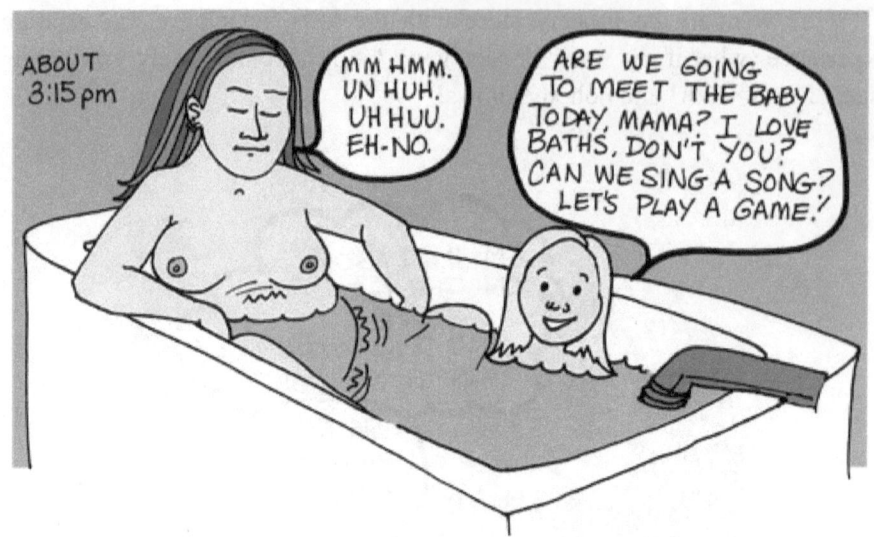

At 4:15 the contractions are more difficult, though I'm exhilarated in between them, but I have a moment in which I really want to throw up. Which excites me even further because everyone agrees that that's a sign that transition is upon you, and this has been so easy and it's almost over!

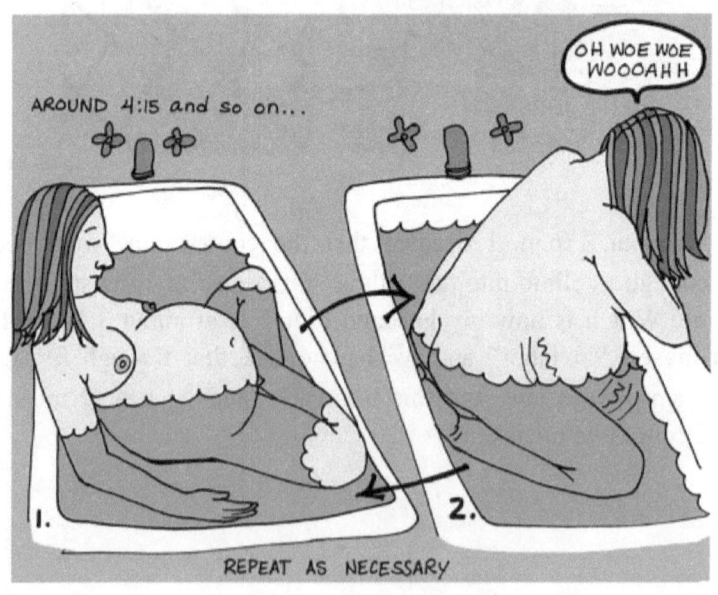

From five to six-ish my thoughtful husband brings in the iPod cued to Eddie Vedder's *Into the Wild* soundtrack. I sing along. Then I get cold but can't be bothered to add more hot water so I decide to get out. The contractions are slamming me at this point and I can feel them all in the lower back.

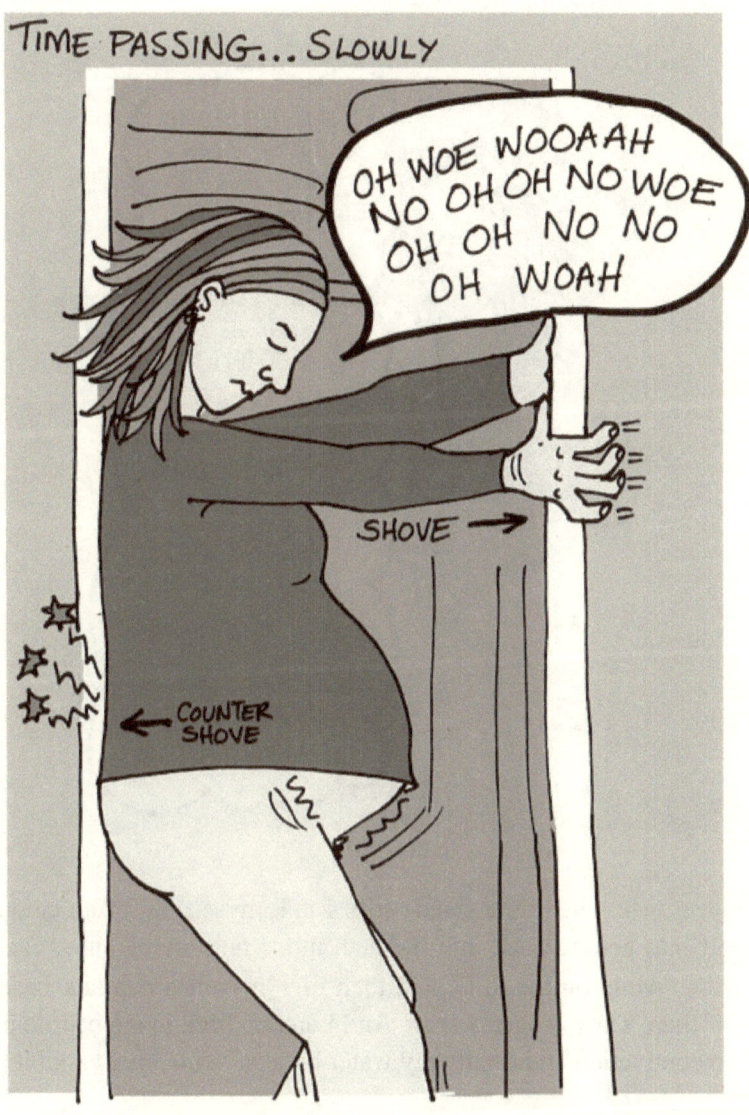

Six-ish and so forth and so on… The contractions are coming one after another and all I want to do is lie down, but I found that if I shove my lower back into the door frame of the closet I can feel a little relief, but man, all I want to do is lie down in between them and the bed is so far away and getting back up to the door jam is so awful and I begin to despair.

My knowing husband, reading my mind, begins to appear during contractions to give me a lower back massage.

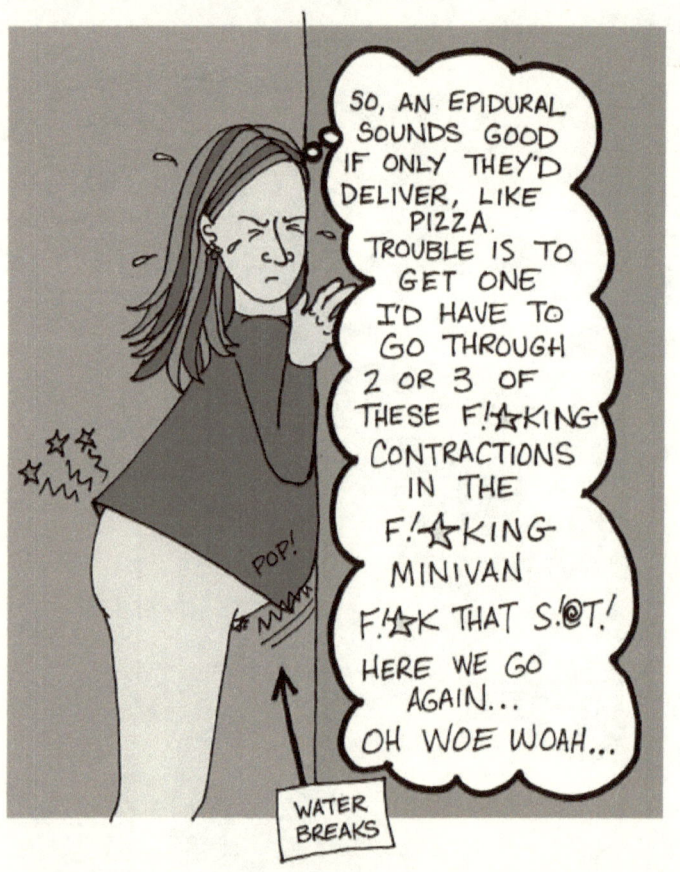

Seven-ish, when time stands still. I talk myself out of an epidural. I talk myself into getting back into the bath tub. I talk myself into "checking my progress" while on the toilet and then give myself a pep talk because I can't tell if there's any progress at all. And I end up back in the bedroom for a doozy of a contraction and finally my water breaks. Something tangible!

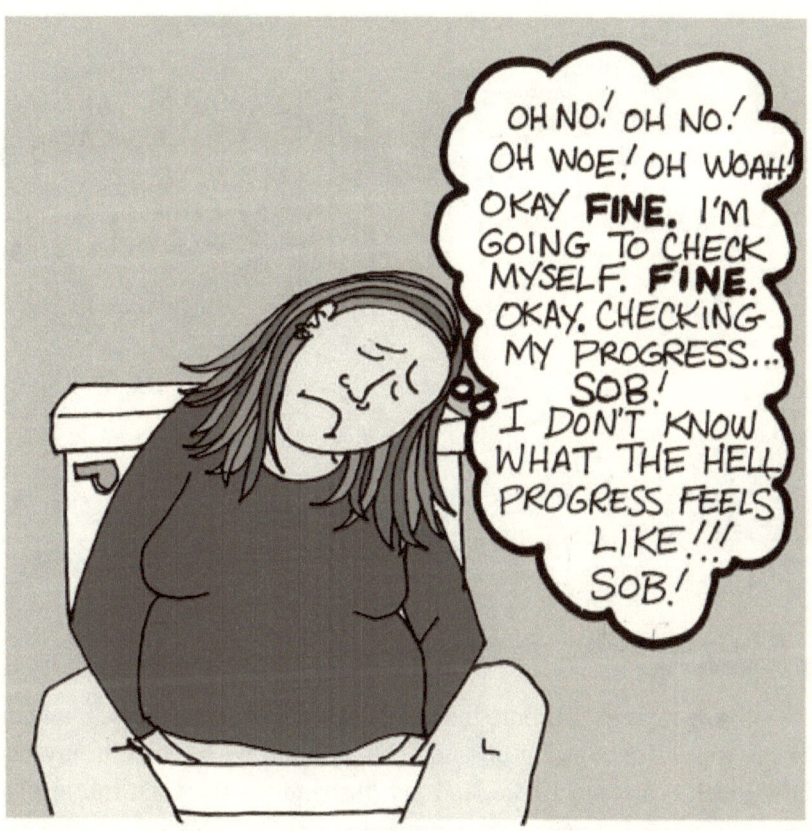

I go back into the bathroom because the toilet seems like the most comfortable place to be, but because I have filled the bathtub with steamy water, it's also hot. Horribly hot, sweat-pouring-down-your-face hot. I wonder if my husband can open the window, but I am seriously, loudly vocalizing through all the contractions (who am I kidding? I'm vocalizing like a banshee almost constantly now!) so I decide to go into the bedroom again.

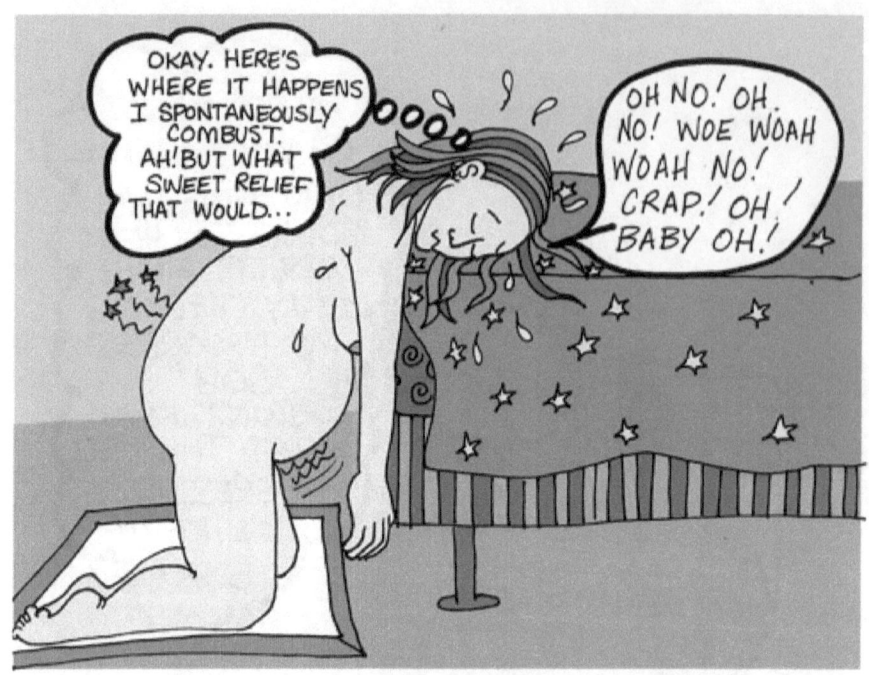

I throw my top half onto the bed in absolute despondency, I am at the end of my rope. I'm carrying on and sobbing and Oy! the pain in my back, and how much more can I take, and my husband continues to rub my back and I have two huge contractions right there and then *pushing*! Immediately. No lull at all. I'm pushing! I thank the heavens and stars and a few choice deities and start to push like crazy wanting to get the baby out. Right. Now.

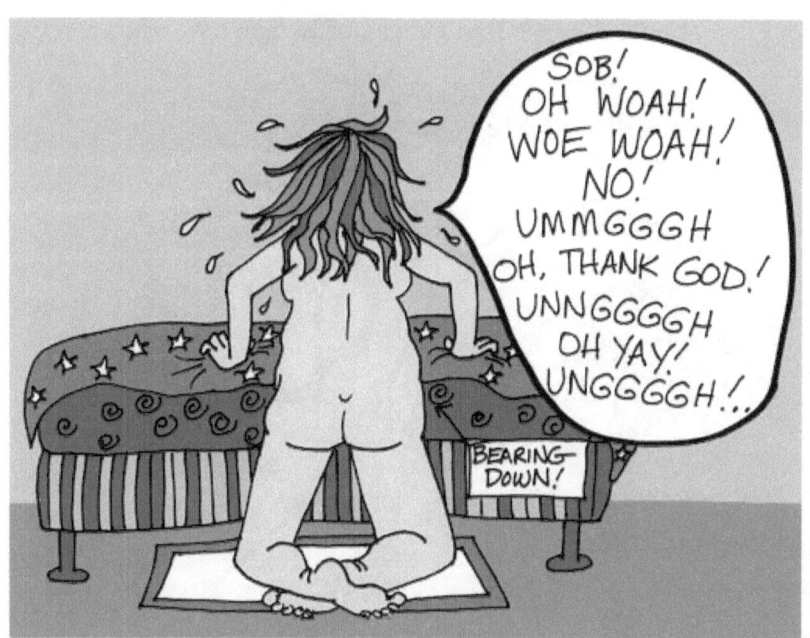

No "breathing the baby out" for me. (I do remember to put my hand back there to support my perineum a bit while I shove like mad though.) I have three pushing contractions, the burning ring of fire, and feel the squirming legs turning the baby (up surprisingly high) and then plop! out onto the towels right between my knees where I'm kneeling.

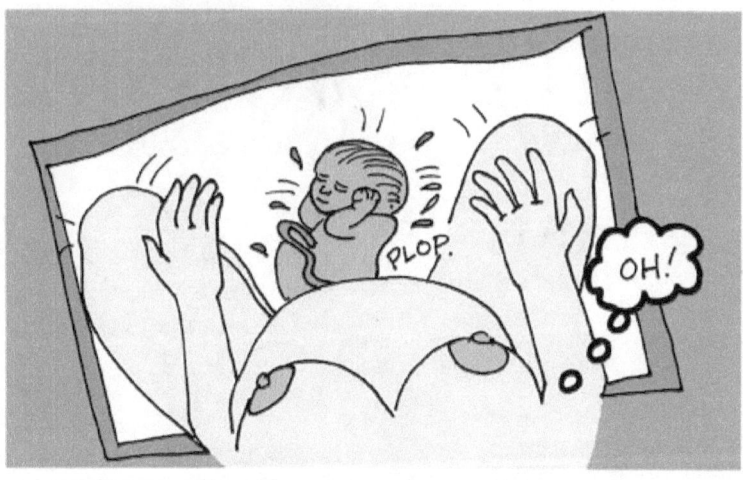

8:15 p.m. A boy! We called the girls in to see their new brother.

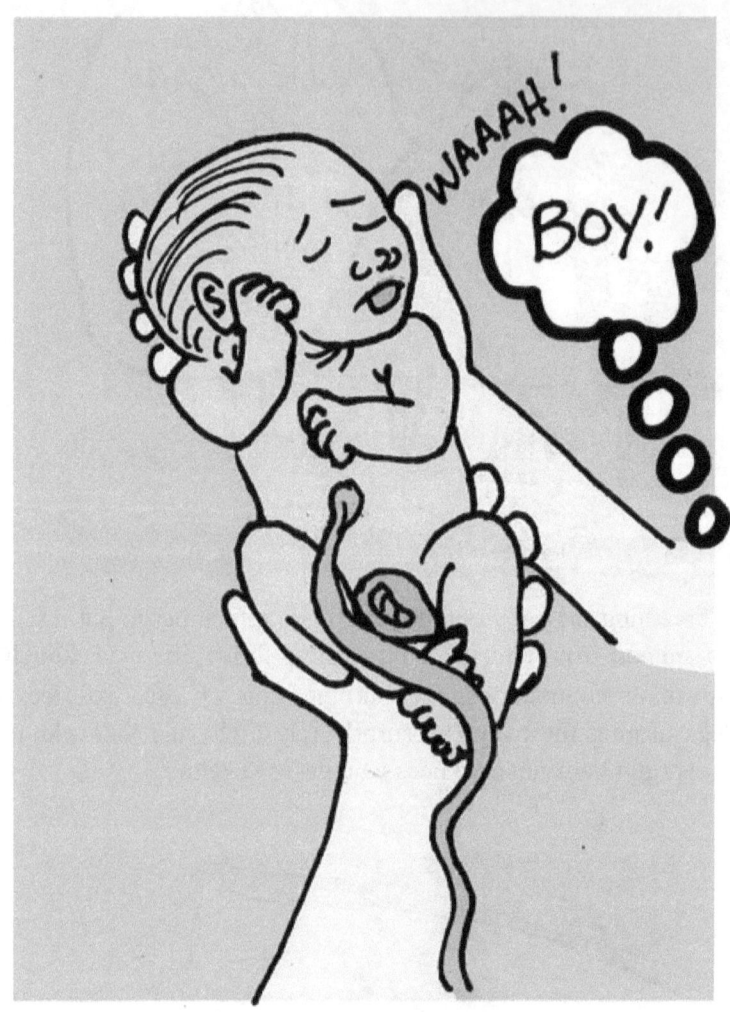

He was gurgly, so I put his bottom higher than his top until he sneezed.

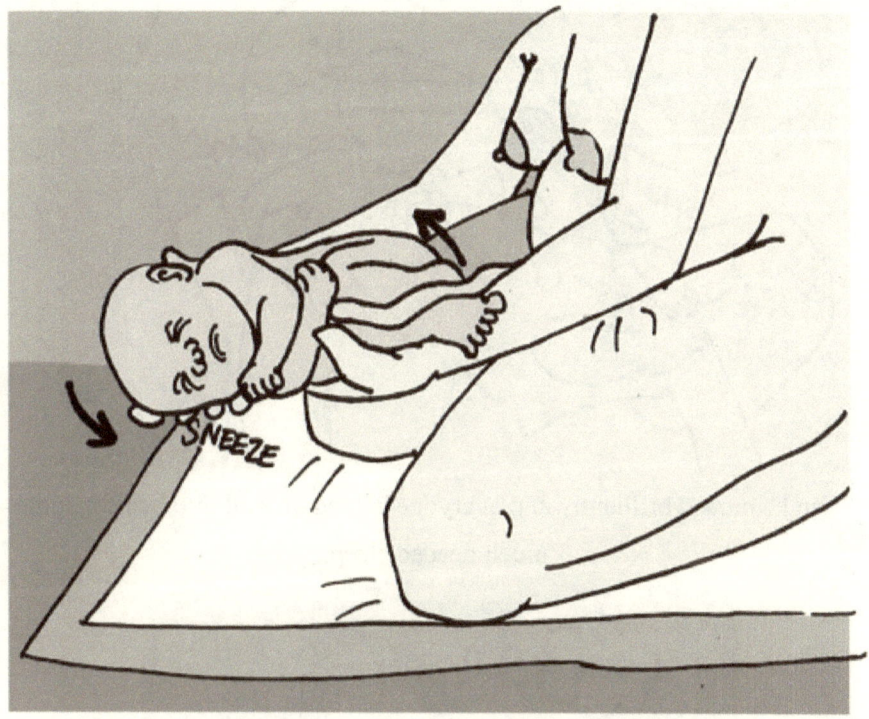

He pinked up perfectly, and after about 20 minutes the placenta unceremoniously plopped out. We tied the cord with an embroidery thread of jaunty orange, and my middle daughter volunteered to do the honors and make the cut.

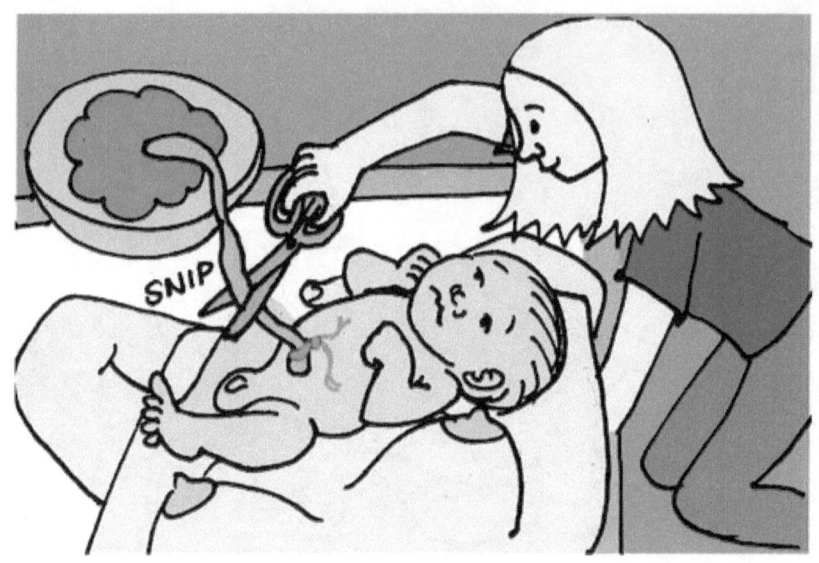

Then he nursed brilliantly and everyone helped me roll into bed for some
much needed sleep.

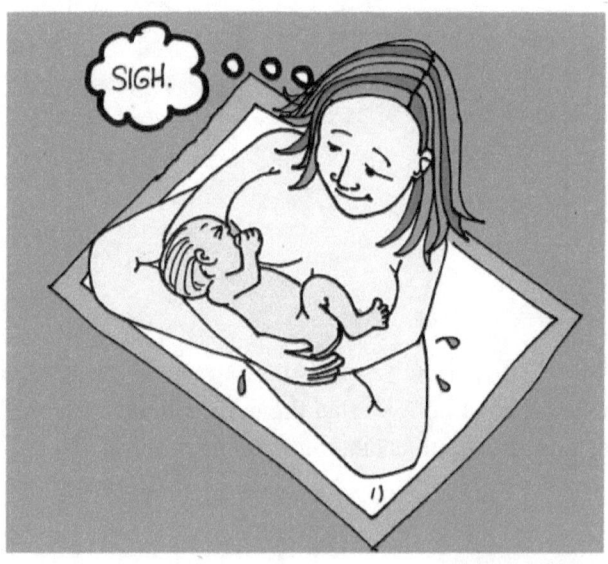

Meet My Friends

Poppy Street-Heywood is a devoted wife and busy mom of 4 homeschooled daughters. She is also a midwife and perpetual student hoping to one day achieve true know-it-all status.

Andi Starr lives in America's Heartland with her soon-to-be embalmer husband, two (almost three!) crazy kids, and two equally crazy cats. When she's not on one of her 'militant hippy' tirades, she's either knitting, sewing, reading, gardening, or cooking good food for her fabulous friends.

Erika Devine is a devoted mother of two boys (both breastfeeding at ages 2 and 5). She can be found at festivals drinking chai tea and at Stonehenge drinking gin and tonic. Her friends joke that she should wear a badge that says, "Ask me about breastfeeding...'cos I'm going to tell you about it anyway"

Talitha L. S. Sherman is the full time homeschooling mother of Kira, Sadie, Hazel, and Theophrastus, and a part time childbirth educator, belly dancer, La Leche League Leader, artist, and Hippo Goddess.

Amy Bell is a birth activist and following the path to doula; while breastfeeding, pampering, and otherwise generally maintaining the family unit; and juggling her commitment to the Ruby Bloomers Women's Circus. She wants to retire to a secluded bush property to write and illustrate books. Adam is a sparky (electrician), and an environmentalist, and an Aboriginal (Wiradjuri) man, striving to find his place in the crazy world of consumerism. Adam also volunteers as a Rural Firefighter.

Heather Farley is the mother of a beautiful girl and hopes to be the mother of many more. She is most well-known for arranging the nurse-in at Facebook Headquarters in December 2008. She feels we need to have more books about strong women, so she hopes to write biographies in the future. In the meantime, she knits and plays all day.

Naomi Sand is the whacko (because she doesn't feel that "crunchy" or "alternative" say enough, when so many of *those* moms have regular supermarket cleaners under their sinks and SUVs that get 10 mpg) mom to two intentionally conceived and very much wanted girls. She likes to find out about doing things in a way that is spiritual and honors the planet and is always open to new wisdom. So, of course, her older girl nursed for close to six years and still cosleeps whenever she pleases and her younger one cosleeps and nurses past her fourth birthday. Her whole whacko unschooled family eats organic food and always focuses on minimizing their carbon footprint.

Lynn Grabowski is a stay-at-home mom to three life-loving unschooled boys. She lives on a six acre farm in southern Ohio with pastured Icelandic sheep, angora rabbits, free range chickens and a happy kitten. Her current goals are toward an organic, sustainable, and eco-friendly lifestyle. She enjoys spending time with the kids, knitting, crocheting, spinning, and watching bad reality TV with her husband.

Mandy Bell is mom to two rambunctious boys who were nursed, cloth-diapered, coslept, and so forth for their all-too-short babyhoods and now enjoy bike rides, video games, all sports, and getting dirty. She's a Kentucky girl living in Ann Arbor, MI, while her husband gets a PhD. She is currently an apprentice midwife, but considering the multitude of ways she can work to make the world a better place.

Lauren F. Jackson is a cloth-diapering, co-sleeping, breastfeeding, babywearing, freebirthing, lactivist, intactivist, crunchy granola stay-at-home earth mommy. She's a crazy Pagan married to a straight-laced Catholic since 1998, and her household is ruled by two wildling boys and five idiosyncratic cats. She spends her free time watching HGTV, doing DIY projects, decorating her home, thrift shopping, bellydancing, and fire-eating.

Jess Urwin is a happily married, homeschooling, homebirthing/ucing mama to five wonderful little people. She is working part time right now but can't wait to be a stay at home mama again. She lives in rural Iowa and dreams of living somewhere more crunchy.

Heather Hawkes is a mother of five wonderful children, married to her main man for 18 years. She is a part time RN and a full-time mama. She loves home cooking, homeschooling and home birthing...She likes doing things at home. She is very interested in breastfeeding, childbirth, permaculture, community building, and alternative energy. At press time, Heather is trying for baby number 6!

Jen Holland is an American expat in Sydney, and she lives with her Aussie husband and three unschooled children. She is passionate about good food and is the owner of The Laughing Planet Baking Company, a whole foods bakery.

Amber Magnolia spends most of her time mothering, some of her time reading all kinds of books about all kinds of things, and the rest of her time blogging about herbs, food, culture, community, and evolution at www.nourishedmother.com.

Janet Fraser is the National Convenor of the Australian homebirth network, Joyous Birth. http://www.joyousbirth.info/ She divides her time between two children, a laptop and life. She is a voice of reason in a woman-hating, birth-hating world, and after the resounding success of Homebirth Awareness Year in 2008 is promoting Birth Trauma Awareness Year in 2009.

Jamie Marr Castillo is a Southern California mama of three children ages 4, 2, and brand new. She has chosen to birth all of her children at home simply because she is healthy and finds homebirth to be a lot easier in terms of freedom and comfort measures and just being able to tune in to the body. She wants every woman to know that they have the power inside of them to birth.

Christy Lindsey is happily married to her soulmate, Matt. She is mom and stepmom to four sons and must really like testosterone. She loves Jesus and enjoys hanging out with her crew, reading, homeschooling, gardening, dancing, massaging, the great outdoors, and listening to Matt play guitar.

Rebekah W, her husband Christopher, and their son Francis live in western Arkansas and operate a graphic/web design/printing company. They enjoy many aspects of natural living and spend much of their spare time reading and traveling.

Jennifer S. Bax is the harried mother of three free-range, unschooled children, a birth advocate and VBACtivist, a trained anthropologist, and an aspiring member of the "knit-your-own-yogurt" crowd. After surviving two cesareans (one arguably necessary, the other most assuredly not), she became an RN in self-defense, and now works on a busy mother/baby unit, supporting new families and hoping that the occasional well-placed suggestion to "please enjoy your baby" hits home for some. She has an extensive online social network (mostly for birth issues), a demanding job, a lot of misplaced guilt and anger, and a profound sleep deficit.

Sara "Seraf" Fones is a twenty-something single mom of two Ohioans. When not nursing in public, she is generally found in the company of octogenarians.

Martha Ellen Cahalan is a mother of many (six, at last count). Her children are homeschooled. They keep her very busy.

Melissa Bellemare is a full-time unschooling mama living in the province of Québec. Her passions are cooking, photography, blogging under the pseudonym of "paxye" and being a Natural parenting/living advocate. She has had three very different births including one UC (unassisted childbirth) and is planning a second UC in January of 2010. Most of all, she loves to laugh and learn through life with her three energetic boys and amazing husband.

Stephanie Whalen lives with her husband and four children (three girls and one surprise baby boy!) in Las Vegas, NV. The youngest two were born at home, unassisted. She enjoys writing stories, taking photos, and watching her children grow and learn every day.

Kelly Silliman and her husband Tom own Sweet Dog Farm, a sustainable agriculture (ad)venture in central Virginia, where they live with their three amazing homeschooled daughters and their newborn son, all born at home. They also own The Dance Barn, a studio that offers classes in ballet, tap, jazz, modern and ballroom dance to children of all ages and adults. Kelly secretly loves Jelly Bellies and can tie shoelaces in a bow with her toes.

Tasha Rose-Mirick is a twenty-eight year old stay-at-home and work-at-home mother to two unschooled daughters, and is pregnant with baby number three, due sometime after Thanksgiving but before Yuletide 2008. Together with her husband, she lives a simple Pagan life in the woods of Northern Minnesota, tending chickens, rabbits, dairy and meat goats and organic gardens. She works as a certified doula, is a studying midwife, a bellydancer and an accomplished seamstress.

Valerie Wassergeburt is a firm believer in the ability and right of a woman to birth unassisted. She believes that a woman's body can birth most efficiently when the woman is in a setting where she feels comfortable and when she has no fear of labor, being fully confident in her abilities. She is wife to her loving and supportive husband Jon and mother to her son Nathan. She is caretaker to many chickens, horses, cows, goats, dogs and other creatures of the Earth. In her spare time she reads and writes about subjects empowering towards Unassisted Pregnancy/Unassisted Childbirth, and attachment parenting. She enjoys drawing and creating with her hands as well as growing her garden and her long hair! She believes in holistic and organic approaches to living and passionately shares her views with those around her.

Kelli Cymraes Lincoln is a radical unschooling mama to four homebirthed beauties, living in the gorgeous Sierra Nevadas. She divides her time between exploring and learning with the family and being creative with her other baby, DancingGoddessDolls.com. She tries to get out of washing dishes as often as possible.

Rebekah Costello is a happily married mother of two little girls living in central Maryland. She is an aspiring midwife and a doula and is patiently expecting her third child any time now!

The Editing Process

The birth stories collected in this book have been edited for space considerations and for ease of reading.

My theory is that we should have two stories for every birth, the first would be the one we write just after the birth, it's a blow-by-blow account with the minutiae of details that you would want when you reread it to yourself 20 years later. Account for everything now, for when your memory escapes you later.

The second birth story should be the one you share, with the minutiae taken out and the universal truths kept in; so that when a pregnant mother comes across your story she can place herself in it, and not have to slog through the retelling of 'Aunt Edna's mastery of the PB and J' between the contractions.

Here's some examples of things I might have removed:

- The Beginning—The weeks worth of contractions (or more!) that led up to active birth. They were felt at school, church, and shopping, and were full of extra characters and random conversations, I removed most of them and started the story at active birth.
- The End—the sum up, the weight, length, height of the baby, the days of nursing bliss following, and the statements that compare this birth to all the

births that have gone before. For the most part I removed it and ended the story just after the placenta appeared.

- The excess cast of characters—beyond the mother and the husband, the other actors are just bit-part players, to save space and interest they were removed if possible.
- Kids—if the story is bogged down in the details of where the kids are, what they were watching on t.v., and how they felt about the birth, they were heartbreakingly removed.
- Long loving compliments to the amazing wondrousness that is our husband. We all know he's great, but birth is your day to shine, he can get a compliment to his awesomeness in print when he pushes a baby out of his wazoo. Long loving compliments to ourselves, on the other hand, will appear in italics. And bold.
- Really, anything that doesn't further the story, if a sentence about Uncle Joe calling you during your birth to tell you what was on America's Talent Show last night can be removed without hurting the continuity of the story, it was removed.

For the authors, this amount of editing is a somewhat brutal process. Birth is one of the defining moments of our lives, and so the details stick with us, they seem crucial to the story, and any removal of them can feel like we're not telling the whole story. But, to get all of these awesome stories into print, and make room for the comics too, editing had to happen. If you'd like to see some of the stories in their original form, some even have photos, a few exist on the web (where space is not a consideration).

Links can be found online at: www.simplygivebirth.com.

Acknowledgements

I want to thank Mara Donahoe, for listening to me yammer on and on about this project, for offering to help, for reading all of the birth stories with me, and then for being so understanding when my control-freak side emerged, and I did it all by myself anyway. Thank you, you're a true and gracious friend.

A huge thank you to Kathleen McKernan-Whitfield for checking this baby for typos. I always knew you were a good editor and then you returned this covered in red marks, and I do mean covered. For gently reminding me that the period goes *inside* quotation marks, I'm ever grateful. And thanks, Deborah Markus, for being called into typo-check service at our homeschool parkday and rising to the occasion, again.

I also want to thank Isobel, Fiona, and Gwynnie Dowdee, for being so helpful and understanding as I wrote and edited, and edited, and edited, this book. I know it seemed endless, but like I promised, it did end.

I definitely want to thank all of the mothers who sent in birth stories, the ones that were chosen and the ones that weren't. Thank you for letting me read them, and subsequently giving me baby fever, and making Ean possible.

And a big giant heap of love to my husband for letting me.

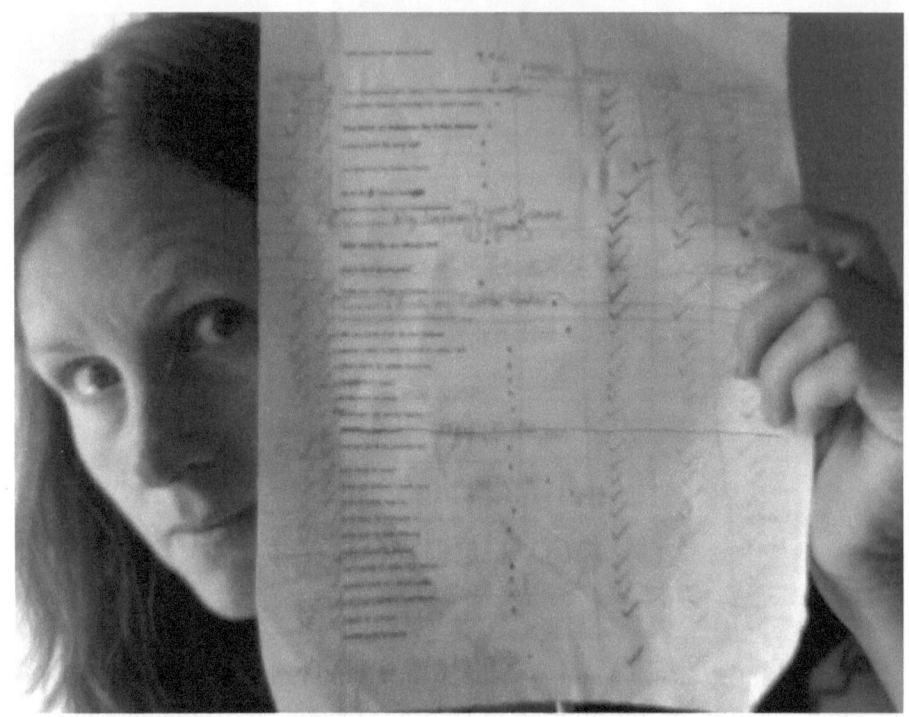

Me with the list of authors, trying like crazy to organize this book!

Heather Cushman-Dowdee is the creator of the comics Hathor the Cowgoddess and Mama is..., She's the crunchy-urban mother of four precociously exuberant children and happily together (twenty years!) with an ocean-loving man. She divides her time between unschooling the kids, breastfeeding the baby, passing out kisses and hugs, expounding on her belief system, reading on the beach, going for long walks, drawing with magic markers, and staring at a computer. She is fighting a losing battle to be a neo-luddite.

A year ago, when Heather first collected these birth stories, she asked the mothers for an author blurb. This was the example she gave them: "Heather Cushman-Dowdee is a superior mother of three who bides her time between massaging her husband feet, changing diapers, and lifting high-rise buildings over her head. She's the author of three books and an almost daily comic about the philosophy of world booboos and big bubble theories." And that's all still mostly true, just more kids.

www.ingramcontent.com/pod-product-compliance
Lightning Source LLC
Chambersburg PA
CBHW061258280526
45784CB00002B/805